New Directions in Critical Public Health

W0036944

In an era where debates about public health research, policy, and practice are central to the wider socio-political discourse, this invaluable volume brings together key themes from the last 15 years of critical scholarship in and of public health.

The book provides both empirical examples and the conceptual tools for rethinking the role of public health in society, challenging the familiar biomedicalized and individualized discourse that has dominated throughout the COVID-19 pandemic. Divided into nine chapters, it covers key topics such as complex systems of health determinants, evidence-making in public health, and the role of corporate actors and philanthropists. Reframing the field through local and global political lenses, *New Directions in Critical Public Health: Health in Turbulent Times* also integrates interdisciplinary perspectives to provide a truly holistic overview of this rapidly evolving area.

It will interest not only students and scholars of public health and the health sciences more widely, but also those in the fields of sociology, political and development studies, and economics.

Lindsay McLaren is Professor of Population and Public Health at the University of Calgary, Canada; Research Associate at the Canadian Centre for Policy Alternatives (National Office); and Co-Editor of the *Journal of Critical Public Health*.

Judith Green is Professor of Sociology in the Centre for Cultures and Environments of Health and the Department of Social and Political Sciences, Philosophy, and Anthropology, University of Exeter, UK, and Co-Editor of the *Journal of Critical Public Health*.

Ronald Labonté is Professor Emeritus in the School of Epidemiology and Public Health, University of Ottawa, Canada; a member of the global People's Health Movement's Steering Council; and Co-Editor-in-Chief of *Globalization and Health*.

New Directions in Critical Public Health

Health in Turbulent Times

Lindsay McLaren, Judith Green, and Ronald Labonté

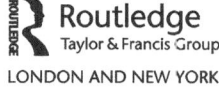

Routledge
Taylor & Francis Group

LONDON AND NEW YORK

Designed cover image: Getty

First published 2026
by Routledge
4 Park Square, Milton Park, Abingdon, Oxon OX14 4RN

and by Routledge
605 Third Avenue, New York, NY 10158

Routledge is an imprint of the Taylor & Francis Group, an informa business

First edition published by Routledge 2008

British Library Cataloguing-in-Publication Data
A catalogue record for this book is available from the British Library

ISBN: 978-1-041-10365-3 (hbk)
ISBN: 978-1-032-35480-4 (pbk)
ISBN: 978-1-003-65465-0 (ebk)

DOI: 10.4324/9781003654650

Typeset in Times New Roman
by Newgen Publishing UK

Contents

Figures

Author biographies

Lindsay McLaren is Professor of Population and Public Health at the University of Calgary, Canada; Research Associate at the Canadian Centre for Policy Alternatives (National Office); and Co-Editor of the Journal of Critical Public Health. Her research interests include social determinants and political economy of health.

Judith Green is Professor of Sociology in the Centre for Cultures and Environments of Health and the Department of Social and Political Sciences, Philosophy, and Anthropology, University of Exeter, UK, and Co-Editor of the Journal of Critical Public Health. Her research interests include the sociology of health and medicine; methodology; and the links between transport, mobility, and health.

Ronald Labonté is Professor Emeritus in the School of Epidemiology and Public Health, University of Ottawa, Canada; a member of the global People's Health Movement's Steering Council; and Co-Editor-in-Chief of Globalization and Health. His research interests are in promoting health equity from local to global scales.

Acknowledgements

We wish to acknowledge the Editorial Collective of the *Journal of Critical Public Health* for their support and solidarity. We extend particular thanks to past co-editors Kirsten Bell and Robin Bunton. Finally, we owe a huge thanks to Chelsea Cox for help in preparing this manuscript.

Introduction

This book started out as an intended second edition of *Critical Perspectives in Public Health* (Green and Labonté 2008). That original volume brought together influential articles from the journal *Critical Public Health*, contextualized by analytical introductory chapters, with the intent to examine "the contemporary roles of 'critical voices' in public health research and practice from a range of disciplines and contexts" (from the back cover).

A great deal has changed since that 2008 publication, including, as we describe below, the landscape of scholarly publishing. These changes have inevitably shaped the current volume, including the decision to produce a stand-alone work of analytic chapters rather than a second edited edition. Yet, while much has changed, the importance of critical public health scholarship has not; indeed, we assert that the need for critical perspectives has, if anything, grown since that time. To introduce this volume, we thus begin by discussing the notion of critical public health – what it is and why it remains important. We then situate the volume within socio-political context, including very significant shifts in global political economy with immense implications for the public's health and for critical scholarship in public health. We conclude this introduction chapter with an overview of the chapters that follow.

What is critical public health and why does it (continue to) matter?

While both 'critical' and 'public health' are contested concepts, that does not preclude articulating contours that shape and ground this volume.

First, what do we mean by *critical*? The synthesis by Green and Labonté (2008) provides an excellent foundation. They begin with the work of Harvey (1990), who articulated that critical perspectives involve:

> deconstructing taken-for-granted concepts and theoretical relationships by asking how these taken-for-granted elements actually relate to wider oppressive structures and how these structures legitimate and conceal their oppressive mechanisms.
>
> (p. 32)

DOI: 10.4324/9781003654650-1

Labonté et al. (2005) helpfully added that critical perspectives serve to both *uncover* and *challenge*; that is, they carry an obligation not only "to uncover how specific social structures, in their political and historical contexts, both construct and recreate conditions that threaten the health of populations or of particular groups within those populations" (Green and Labonté 2008, p. 4) but also to challenge those structures and seek the "reconstruction of social, economic and political relations along emancipatory lines" (Green and Labonté 2008; Labonté et al. 2005, p. 10) Several scholars (e.g. Krieger 2000; Labonté et al. 2005; Schrecker 2022) have emphasized the inherently normative nature of critical perspectives in public health, where one must 'take sides'. Krieger (2000), for example, argues for a "passionate epistemology" which is "at once critical, rigorous, humble and partisan" on the side of those who disproportionately suffer from harmful systems and structures (pp. 287–288).

While recognizing that critical perspectives in public health are not monolithic and "do not necessarily speak in unison" (p. 5), Green and Labonté (2008) offer a very helpful heuristic in the form of a critical voice *for* public health and a critique *of* public health. A critical voice *for* public health means a stance for uncovering the health-damaging effects of particular social structures, in their political and historical contexts, and challenging those structures. Speaking to the normative element, this includes the obligation to act as advocates when certain values, such as the vested interests of business, trump others such as health and equity (Green and Labonté 2008). A critique *of* public health, on the other hand, involves asking difficult questions about our field's successes and failures and constantly questioning our own assumptions. This involves reflection, from a place of humility, about the ways in which we benefit from, and are complicit in, the status quo, both as individuals (who may be well paid professionals with secure employment) and as a field (Green and Labonté 2008).

Public health is consistently defined as something along the lines of the art and science of preventing disease and promoting health through organized efforts of society (Acheson 1988; Canadian Public Health Association n.d.). This definition encompasses some core features which theoretically distinguish it from other institutionalized aspects of 'health', such as clinical medicine. These distinguishing features include a population-level lens and an 'upstream' focus on why people get sick in the first place, and inequitably so (McLaren et al. 2024). The extent to which these core features are realized is strongly influenced, or indeed constrained, by a constellation of intersecting historical, ideological, epistemological, and professional factors which often – and increasingly – result in a medicalized, decontextualized, and technical version of public health in education, research, policy, and practice spaces (e.g. McLaren and Mykhalovskiy 2024); these dynamics are key concerns of critical public health scholars. It is important for us to be explicit about our intent, in this volume, to instead embrace a version of public health as social activism. This is consistent with the 2008 volume, which noted inspiration from Rudolph Virchow, who, throughout his 19th-century career, "saw no distinction between being a health professional and a social activist" (Green and Labonté 2008, p. xiv). An alternatively worded, but highly consistent, stance that we embrace in this work is a social democratic public health, which we briefly discuss in Chapter 3.

Significantly, however, an activist stance is not tension-free. As Green and Labonté (2008) argue, "we cannot make sense of public health purely in its own terms" (p. 9). Public health has much to do with the state as a co-creator of conditions of well-being. Yet, where one draws the line between the state as a site of social empowerment, and one of repression, is blurry and contested. If, as Green and Labonté (2008) ask, public health is partly about regulating our social world towards some collective good, which is how Virchow viewed it, what is 'good'? How is it to be governed into existence? And who decides? These questions, Green and Labonté (2008) argue, are at the core of our field and must be problematized.

These dynamics underpin the presence of what can be seen as two 'camps' within critical public health scholarship. On the one hand, there are those, often situated in the political economy space, who are focused on 'macro'-forces such as neoliberalism and on illuminating the impact of those macro-forces on health. On the other hand, there are those, often situated in anthropology, Science and Technology Studies (STS), and postmaterialist scholarship, who actively resist the position of assuming the existence of macro-level forces and instead emphasize the need to explain how power is made locally. This can potentially open up new ways of doing health, human flourishing, and social justice. Both perspectives are very much concerned with politics, but the terms of engagement are very different: while the former group of scholars accepts, to at least some extent, the existence of macro-forces and moves on from there, the latter scholars would instead engage in ways that are rooted in local and contingent enactments. That is, those latter perspectives are more directed at the micro-level and the material, as well as human, actors that come together to 'do' health.

An excellent illustration of the two 'camps', and, we argue, their complementarity, is a 2021 special issue of *Critical Public Health* focused on public health activism. In the accompanying editorial, Campbell and Cornish (2021) define critical public health activism "in terms of collective efforts to redistribute power in ways that create more health-enabling social environments in conditions of social inequality" (p. 130). The collection of papers includes, first of all, important examples of traditional forms of social activism, which the editors summarize as "a public battle between the powerful and the powerless, conceived of as clearly identifiable groups" (p. 6). Papers in this theme, which align more with the 'macro'-stance in critical public health, illustrate "both the hopes and potentials, but also the very severe limitations of, social movement approaches from one context to another in the current socio-political climate" (p. 128). One example, by Egan et al. (2021), concerned a charity initiative in the UK that funded grassroots members of disadvantaged communities towards improving their built environment, ultimately highlighting the impossibility of expecting collective action by charities and small residents' communities in the context of decimating austerity (Campbell and Cornish 2021).

Another set of papers in the special issue, which align more with the 'local, contingent networks' stance of critical public health, illustrate "novel or previously unrecognized forms of public health activism", which "open up completely different ways of thinking about the nature of collective agency and social change" (p. 128). These papers are diverse, but one example by Clinch (2021) considers, in the context of planetary devastation, the work of volunteer environmental stewards in rural northern England and celebrates their small-scale efforts in "enacting a radical determination to imagine and develop less destructive ways of living together" (Campbell and Cornish 2021, p. 130). In a similar vein, Martinez-Lacabe (2021) considers how gay British men at risk of HIV were able to collectively harness the logic of the market to develop a 'grey market', which facilitated access to medical treatments in a way that bypassed state and medical authorities, thus disrupting a traditional ('macro')-understanding of activism as opposition to the neoliberal status quo.

Overall, the special issue illustrates what Campbell and Cornish (2021) describe as a "need for radical expansion of what public health activists should regard as evidence for redistribution of power" (p. 126), noting that, in contrast to the traditional (and colonial, as argued by Gumbonzvanda et al. 2021) version of activism as "visible social change via organized resistance" (p. 128), marginalized communities constantly engage in far quieter and less obvious forms of redistribution in ways that are often very effective in supporting their health and well-being. Campbell and Cornish's call for "radical expansion" is consistent with the notion of *prefigurative action* that we pick up on in the Conclusion chapter of this volume.

The journal *Critical Public Health* had, up to December 2023 (see below), always held the uneasiness of the two 'camps'. While not always straightforward to navigate, we ultimately believe that this is a strength of the field. Indeed, as Green and Labonté (2008) argued, while "playing the role of the advocate and learning the arts of politics are legitimate roles for public health activists, ... critical voices also need to be penetrating, rather than unquestioningly championing those policies which appear to be 'good things'" (p. 6). Thus, while not without tension, these two stances can be seen as complementary, and they make for a robust forum indeed for discussion and debate around the immensely important task of uncovering and challenging (as per Labonté et al. 2005) harmful social structures.

Situating critical public health in socio-political context

The 2008 publication date of the earlier volume (Green and Labonté 2008) is significant and merits some brief discussion. This was the time of the global financial crisis and a pinnacle – at that time – of the disastrous experiment of global neoliberal political economics. The immense significance of that paradigm for health equity (e.g. Labonté and Stuckler 2016) has led to it figuring prominently in critical public health scholarship, as discussed especially in Chapter 6 of this volume.

While the 2008 crisis shattered the credibility of neoliberalism, the paradigm persisted, leading Canadian progressive economist Osberg (2021) to describe the post-2008 political economy as one of "Zombie Neo-liberalism" (p. 7), because no coherent alternative had yet emerged to replace it. While the 2008 crisis itself presented a key opportunity to advance a new political economic paradigm, corporations and their allies – including in governments across the political spectrum – doubled down to obstruct changes to the policies that caused the crisis in the first place. Likewise, the COVID-19 pandemic, which laid bare the profound gaps and injustices built into our public services and supports and decision-making structure, offered an important opportunity to advance a more equity-centred political economy; once again, however, we largely returned to business as usual (McLaren et al. 2023; see also Taher et al. 2025).

At the time of writing this Introduction chapter, the USA had recently elected a tyrant for their president, "an authoritarian strongman, and now convicted felon, who is more articulate in his disdain for others than in his policy positions or goals for his presidency" (Antin and Hunt 2025, p. 1). Neoliberalism is likely dead, but contrary to the glimmer of hope embedded in the 'zombie' concept, we now appear to be in something much worse. We pick this up in the Conclusion chapter.

What is the role for critical public health in this very uncertain context? Green and Labonté (2008) reflected on this question in the 2008 context, ultimately concluding that despite some promising trends such as increasing attention by governments to social determinants of health and of public participation in the wake of the 2008 release of the World Health Organization (WHO) Commission on Social Determinants of Health (CSDH)'s final report (CSDH 2008), critical public health's 'job' is far from done. This remains true in 2025, and indeed, the chasm between the mainstream, on the one hand, and a radical agenda embodied in critical perspectives, on the other, now feels even greater than in 2008. As just one example, with respect to growing mainstream attention to potentially radical concepts like social determinants of health, critical scholarship has identified a new kind of denialism where the language is invoked but in a way that is downstream, sanitized, and divorced from its roots in power and politics, thus missing – or co-opting – the point entirely (see Chapter 4).

Speaking to the enduring importance of critical perspectives in public health is recent work analysing mainstream public health's engagement with political economy in the Canadian context. Based on an analysis of six historical volumes from the 115-year history of the *Canadian Journal of Public Health (CJPH)*, each selected from a period corresponding to key economic circumstances, McLaren and Mykhalovskiy (2024; see also Labonté, 2024) drew three key conclusions. First, they found only a slim historical foundation for public health engagement with the economy overall. Second, they observed a strong and seemingly subconscious allegiance to dominant economic paradigms, despite their incompatibility with addressing root causes of health inequities. Third, they found that even though socio-economic inequalities in health are a long-standing preoccupation of *CJPH* authors, those inequalities are consistently and curiously divorced from their roots in political economic systems. Most relevant to the present discussion, these authors observed that "when economic circumstances and policy environment were especially problematic [for health equity] (e.g. during the Great Depression, and the Neoliberal era), [*CJPH* authors] seemed to retreat even further into economic rationalization, downstream solutions, and fixation on methods" (p. 711).

Another illustration, again in the Canadian context, is evident in some academic institutions where public health, in the current highly chaotic context, has become a nearly unrecognizable pursuit of unproblematized "scientific excellence" at the expense of any meaningful engagement around harmful trends both within and outside of our field (Haines-Saah and McLaren 2023, p. 711).

In other words, there are indications that, when critical engagement for and of public health is most needed, it is most absent, at least in mainstream spaces. Drawing once again on the powerful commentary from the 2008 volume (Green and Labonté 2008), the need for critical voices that "[play] the role of advocate" in a way that is "penetrating, rather than unquestioningly championing those policies which appear to be 'good things'" (p. 6) seems more necessary than ever.

The evolution and impact of a journal

With this context in mind, and in the interest of ending this Introduction on a note of optimism, we describe recent events in the critical public health community that have shaped this volume, including its format. The 2008 edition (Green and Labonté 2008) was an edited volume that brought together important papers published in the journal *Critical Public Health*. In contrast, the current volume comprises authored analytic chapters that synthesise key content published in *Critical Public Health* up to December 2023 (Volume 33, Issue 5) as well as from other sources. We take some space to describe the context for this decision because it is emblematic of the changing context and the role of critical public health in it.

The history of *Critical Public Health* has been described elsewhere (Green and Labonté 2008; Bell et al. 2021; Green et al. 2023). Briefly, the journal started life in 1979 as a newsletter-style product called *Radical Community Medicine*; the name was a partial honorific to Virchow's work and language (Green and Labonté 2008). Early contributors to *Radical Community Medicine* named and discussed issues that we would now consider core to critical perspectives in public health, such as professional power in medicine and its oppressive effects; the need for participatory democracy and meaningful community engagement in public health; and the importance of determinants of health like living and working conditions (Green and Labonté 2008).

From its *Radical Community Medicine* roots, Bell et al. (2021) describe and reflect on the journal's history in the context of the contemporary publishing landscape:

Rebranded [as *Critical Public Health*] in 1990, it became a fully refereed international journal in 1998, distributed by the academic publisher Carfax (see Bunton, 1998; Bunton and Russell, 1997). Because the periodical had been founded by an informal collective rather than an organisation or society, Carfax took formal ownership over the journal. This made sense in 1997 when the arrangement was worked out: profits were marginal, decision-making power remained with the editors, and authors licensed their copyright to the publisher regardless of the ownership structure. However, the late 1990s was a period of dramatic change in scholarly publishing, marked by rapid corporate consolidation.

The ink was barely dry on our contract with Carfax before they were bought out by Routledge, in turn bought out by the Taylor & Francis Group […] who merged with Informa in 2004. This scenario is reasonably common – by 2015, 70% of all social science publications in Web of Science were published by the so-called 'Big Five' publishers: Elsevier, Springer, Taylor & Francis, Wiley-Blackwell, and Sage (Larivière et al., 2015). This consolidation enabled the emergence of 'big deals': the practice of bundling high prestige journals with lower prestige ones and requiring libraries to pay for the full package to access the journals they wanted (Bergstrom et al., 2014). The resultant serials crisis was a critical trigger for the open access movement (Eve, 2013). Yet, while this movement is fundamentally reshaping the scholarly publishing landscape, it has made little dent in the profits of corporate publishers themselves. For example, Taylor & Francis's 2020 operating profit of £216 million (Chandler, 2021), with its 38% profit margin, is one that most companies can only dream of.

(p. 377, reprinted by permission of Informa UK Limited, trading as Taylor & Francis Group, www.tandfonline.com)

Critical Public Health was thus owned and published by Taylor & Francis for several years, and for many of those years, the arrangement was tenable. As described by Green et al. (2023):

For decades, *Critical Public Health* thrived – if at times uncomfortably – as both a home for debate and radical scholarship, curated on behalf of a wider community by the Editorial Board, and a (presumably) profitable commodity for its publisher.

(p. 504)

However, as Green et al. (2023) went on to say,

the uneasy compromise became impossible to hold. Increasingly, we found ourselves unable to maintain the unique niche of the journal in the light of changes to the commercial publishing landscape and their impact on our ability to set the future strategic direction of the journal.

(p. 504)

One key issue concerned a move to open access under an author-pays or article processing charge (APC) model. While supportive of open access as a *concept*, our editorial board was, not surprisingly, concerned that such a shift would risk compounding existing inequalities (Bell et al. 2021). As Bell et al. (2021) point out, critical scholars are those "working from the epistemic margins" (p. 378): early career scholars, independent scholars, and social scientists working in public health contexts are especially vulnerable to being excluded if funds are needed to publish. Moreover, the APC model inevitably reinforces global inequities in knowledge production, compounding exclusion already experienced by scholars outside the global north (Bell et al. 2021; see also Chapter 1 in this volume).

A larger issue concerns the mission of *Critical Public Health* and *Radical Community Medicine* before it, described by Bell et al. (2021) as "an *intellectual project* driven by a concern about the power relations of knowledge production – especially the role of corporate influences, north-south inequalities, and the politics of disciplinarity" (p. 378, emphasis in original). Indeed, at some level, the corporate publishing landscape is simply incompatible with critical scholarship, and it is perhaps predictable that our arrangement with *Critical Public Health* would become "impossible to hold" (Green et al. 2023).

In July of 2023, members of the international Editorial Board of *Critical Public Health* resigned, en masse, from our corporate publishers (Green et al. 2023; Critical Public Health Network n.d.a). We created a new community, non-profit journal, the *Journal of Critical Public Health*, which is published on the Public Knowledge Project – Open Journal System platform. The journal is published by the Critical Public Health Network, whose purpose is to (1) act as an advocate for the critical public health scholarly community; (2) offer a point of contact for public health practitioners interested in social science/humanities in public health; (3) provide a network for information/knowledge exchange for members to enhance research, policy, and education on and for public health; and (4) continue to develop the spirit and commitment to critical public health initiated in *Radical Community Medicine* (Critical Public Health Network n.d.b). Our reasons for establishing a new journal and our vision for that new journal are communicated in the Manifesto published in our first issue (Bunton 2024).

At the time of writing this Introduction chapter, we had just published our third issue (Volume 2, Issue 1, 2025). This demonstrates, at least so far, that community-owned journals can thrive outside the commercial publishing sector and that we have a way to continue "*Radical Community Medicine's* origins … in the need for a space to challenge public health orthodoxies, shifting the centre and breaking new ground (Scott-Samuel 1998), [which was] a mandate continued by *Critical Public Health* (Bell and Green 2015; Bunton 1998)" (Bell et al. 2021, p. 378).

We believe that our new journal provides one small example of the 'uncovering and challenging' health-damaging social structures (Labonté et al. 2005), including the ground-up resistance and organizing that is required to do so.

The chapters ahead

Continuing threads in this Introduction, Chapter 1 considers the political economy of knowledge production, including the dramatic changes to the scholarly publishing landscape that occurred during the mid-late neoliberal period and their implications for critical scholarship in public health. Building on that analysis, Chapter 2 delves deeper into the contested nature of evidence-making for critical public health, discussing critical contributions to rethinking methodology and working towards epistemic justice.

Chapter 3 considers the persistently relevant framework of *medicalization* to describe oppressive forces of medicine and more recent theoretical advancements in the form of *biomedicalization*. Next, consistent with the 'critical voice *for* public health', Chapter 4 synthesizes important work in social and structural determinants of health and health equity, while Chapter 5 considers theoretical advancements drawing on social practice and 'more than human' approaches to health that have gone 'beyond behaviour' in their analyses of how health gets done. This chapter also touches on attending more carefully to the range of effects that public health practices have in the world, such that critiques 'of' public health do not simply denounce but are productive engagements.

Chapters 6 and 7 take a global perspective, situating critical public health scholarship within neoliberal globalization (Chapter 6) and then considering issues of governance and healthy social movement activism (Chapter 7). Finally, Chapter 8 (Conclusion) reflects on the current, highly uncertain, political economic circumstances and its implications for critical public health .

Consistent with the 2008 volume, "it would be impossible to provide a comprehensive collection on critical public health, and we have not attempted to do so" (p. 9). Reflecting the source work published in *Critical Public Health* and allied journals, we have drawn almost entirely on anglophone commentary; this is an imbalance for which we feel discomfort. A short volume cannot do justice to the entire body of scholarship that was published in *Critical Public Health* between 2008 and 2023 and, more recently, the *Journal of Critical Public Health*, and the choice of focus inevitably reflects our own interests, positions and expertise as authors. We have, for instance, emphasized critical scholarship in the political economy space, more so than work by scholars in anthropology, STS, and postmaterialist spaces. However, we trust that this overview provides an introduction to contemporary developments and new directions.

References

Acheson, D. (1988) *Public health in England. Report of the Committee of Inquiry into the future development of the public health function.* London: House of Commons.

Antin, T. and Hunt, G. (2025) 'Left behind again: rural America and the hypocrisy of populism', *Journal of Critical Public Health*, 2(1), pp. 1–5.

Bell, K. and Green, J. (2015) 'Keeping a critical edge: reflections on 25 years as a scholarly journal', *Critical Public Health*, 25(1), pp. 1-3. Available at: https://doi.org/10.1080/09581596.2014.982879

Bell, K. *et al.* (2021) '"Open" relationships: reflections on the role of the journal in the contemporary scholarly publishing landscape', *Critical Public Health*, 31(4), pp. 377–380. Available at: https://doi.org/10.1080/09581596.2021.1958512

Bergstrom, T.C. *et al.* (2014) 'Evaluating big deal journal bundles', *Proceedings of the National Academy of Sciences*, 111(26), pp. 9425–9430. Available at: https://doi.org/10.1073/pnas.1403006111

Bunton, R. (1998) 'Editorial: *Critical Public Health* –an introduction', *Critical Public Health*, 8(1), pp. 3–8. Available at: https://doi.org/10.1080/09581599808409207

Bunton, R. and Editorial Collective (2024) 'Manifesto for a new journal: safeguarding critique in public health', *Journal of Critical Public Health*, 1(1), pp. 1–4. Available at: https://doi.org/10.55016/ojs/jcph.v1i1.78305

Bunton, R. and Russell, J. (1997) 'The limits to epidemiology re-visited', *Critical Public Health*, 7(1–2), pp. 2–6. Available at: https://doi.org/10.1080/09581599708409074

Campbell, C. and Cornish, F. (2021) 'Public health activism in changing times: re-locating collective agency', *Critical Public Health*, 31(2), pp. 125–133. Available at: https://doi.org/10.1080/09581596.2021.1878110

Canadian Public Health Association (n.d.) 'What is public health?' Available at: www.cpha.ca/what-public-health

Chand er, M. (2021) 'Taylor & Francis revenue and profits see marginal drop in 2020', *The Bookseller*, 21 April. Available at: www.thebookseller.com/news/taylor-francis-revenue-and-profits-fall-marginally-2020-1256467

Clinch, M. (2021) 'Environmental stewardship in austere times: nurturing sustainable socio-ecological relations', *Critical Public Health*, 31(3), pp. 245–254. Available at: https://doi.org/10.1080/09581596.2020.1853057

Commission on Social Determinants of Health (2008) *Closing the gap in a generation: health equity through action on the social determinants of health. Final report of the Commission on Social Determinants of Health*. WHO/IER/CSDH/08.1. Geneva: World Health Organization. Available at: www.who.int/publications/i/item/WHO-IER-CSDH-08.1

Critical Public Health Network (n.d.a) 'About the CPHN'. Available at: https://cphn.net/about/.

Critical Public Health Network (n.d.b) 'Journal of Critical Public Health'. Available at: https://cphn.net/journal-of-critical-public-health/

Egan, M. *et al.* (2021) 'Building collective control and improving health through a place-based community empowerment initiative: qualitative evidence from communities seeking agency over their built environment', *Critical Public Health*, 31(3), pp. 268–279. Available at: https://doi.org/10.1080 /09581596.2020.1851654

Eve, M.P. (2013) 'Publication: "The botnet: webs of hegemony/zombies who publish", in Zombies in the Academy (Bristol: Intellect, 2013)', *Martin Paul Eve*, 2 June. Available at: https://doi.org/10.59348/cama3-wj520

Green, J. and Labonté, R. (eds) (2008) *Critical perspectives in public health*. London: Routledge.

Green, J. *et al.* (2023) 'Moving on in uncertain times: a goodbye', *Critical Public Health*, 33(5), pp. 503–505. Available at: https://doi.org/10.1080/09581596.2023.2248797

Gumbonzvanda, N., Gumbonzvanda, F. and Burgess, R. (2021) 'Decolonising the "safe space" as an African innovation: the Nhanga as quiet activism to improve women's health and wellbeing', *Critical Public Health*, 31(2), pp. 169–181. Available at: https://doi.org/10.1080/09581596.2020.1866169

Haines-Saah, R. and McLaren, L. (2023) 'A cautionary tale: university institutes of public health must "walk the talk"', *Canadian Journal of Public Health*, 114(5), pp. 710–713. Available at: https://doi.org/10.17269/s41997-023-00815-z

Harvey, L. (1990) *Critical social research*. London: Unwin Hyman (Contemporary social research series, 21).

Krieger, N. (2000) 'Passionate epistemology, critical advocacy, and public health: doing our profession proud', *Critical Public Health*, 10(3), pp. 287–294. Available at: https://doi.org/10.1080/713658251

Labonté, R. (2024) 'Public health can no longer fence-sit politically', *Canadian Journal of Public Health*, 115(5), pp. 701–704. Available at: https://doi.org/10.17269/s41997-024-00941-2

Labonté, R. and Stuckler, D. (2016) 'The rise of neoliberalism: how bad economics imperils health and what to do about it', *Journal of Epidemiology and Community Health*, 70(3), pp. 312–318. Available at: https://doi.org/10.1136/jech-2015-206295

Labonté, R. *et al.* (2005) 'Beyond the divides: towards critical population health research', *Critical Public Health*, 15(1), pp. 5–17. Available at: https://doi.org/10.1080/09581590500048192

Larivière, V., Haustein, S. and Mongeon, P. (2015) 'The oligopoly of academic publishers in the digital era', *PLOS One*. Edited by W. Glanzel, 10(6), p. e0127502. Available at: https://doi.org/10.1371

Martinez-Lacabe, A. (2021) 'The PrEP response in England: enabling collective action through public health and PrEP commodity activism', *Critical Public Health*, 31(2), pp. 226–234. Available at: https://doi.org/10.1080/09581596.2020.1844152

McLaren, L. *et al.* (2023) 'Towards an equity-centered political economy', *Think Upstream*, 4 December. Available at:_www.policyalternatives.ca/news-research/towards-an-equity-centered-political-economy/

McLaren, L., Juzwishin, D.W.M. and Mendoza, R.V. (2024) *A history of public health in Alberta, 1919–2019*. Calgary, Alberta: University of Calgary Press.

McLaren, L. and Mykhalovskiy, E. (2024) 'Economic policy and public health: insights from the history of the Canadian Journal of Public Health', *Canadian Journal of Public Health*, 115(5), pp. 705–719. Available at: https://doi.org/10.17269/s41997-024-00940-3

Osberg, L. (2021) *From Keynesian consensus to neo-liberalism to the green new deal: 75 years of income inequality in Canada*. Ottawa, ON: Canadian Centre for Policy Alternatives.

Schrecker, T. (2022) 'What is critical about critical public health? Focus on health inequalities', *Critical Public Health*, 32(2), pp. 139–144. Available at: https://doi.org/10.1080/09581596.2021.1905776

Scott-Samuel, A. (1998) 'Editorial: and in the beginning', *Critical Public Health*, 8(1), pp. 9–12. Available at: https://doi.org/10.1080/09581599808409208

Taher, A., Power, E. and Payne, G. (2025) '"You're just invisible and you don't matter at all": the structural violence of the COVID-19 Canada Emergency Response Benefit (CERB)', *Journal of Critical Public Health*, 2(1), pp. 23–39.

1 Political economy of knowledge production

Political economy provides a framework for thinking about health – or anything else – that centres on the way our economy operates, including its embedded social and political structures and relations. The framework foregrounds the inequalities that arise from conflict between actors and groups with different interests and very different levels of power to realize those interests (Chernomas and Hudson 2013; Harvey 2021).

In our current political economic context of neoliberal capitalism (although see the Conclusion chapter of this volume), the imperative of private profit accumulation and the dominance of the business class shape essentially everything, including the distribution of health and its determinants (see also Chapter 6 in this volume). Neoliberalism's commitment to facilitating private investment for supporting a narrow version of economic growth – which manifests as ideologically driven policy approaches such as trade liberalization; deregulation of extractive industries, labour markets, and the finance sector; and austerity and privatization of public services – demonstrably causes harms to the health of people and to the planet on which we all depend. The hegemony of this paradigm, moreover, perpetuates narratives of scarcity, rationality, efficiency, and individualism that are powerful but highly misleading with respect to providing the conditions needed to support well-being and health equity (Chernomas and Hudson 2013; Harvey 2021; Labonté and Stuckler 2016).

As discussed in this chapter, these dynamics have significant implications for knowledge production – that is, scholarly research or knowledge generation, including the processes shaping it. Within public health and beyond, there have long been significant imbalances in what kinds of research topics, perspectives, and methodologies are prioritized, funded, conducted, published, and mobilized; by whom and where; and to what end(s). These imbalances mirror broader systemic inequities, reflecting competing interests between groups with different levels of social, economic, epistemic, disciplinary, professional, and global/colonial/imperial power. They manifest in the dominance of certain perspectives and exclusion or sidelining of others.

Critical scholarship in public health has much to contribute to understanding the political economy of knowledge production in public health and related areas. In

DOI: 10.4324/9781003654650-2

this chapter, we showcase some of the important scholarship that has illuminated how competing interests and power inequities play out in various stages of knowledge production, including research agenda setting, funding, and scholarly publishing. Importantly, a political economy perspective not only offers an analytic frame for understanding current circumstances but also offers ways forward. We thus conclude with some comments around redressing power and politics as they are embedded in knowledge production processes (see also the Introduction chapter of this volume).

Foundations: different perspectives on health and how to understand it

A high-quality introductory textbook on public or population health will hopefully begin by introducing different ways of thinking about health (e.g. Davidson 2019). It may contrast individual-focused approaches, which centre on biomedical or behavioural factors such as genetic predisposition, 'lifestyle' behaviours, and access to medical care, with population-level structural or political economic approaches. Embedded in these different approaches are substantively different theories or explanations about the causes of poor health, appropriate ways to understand it (epistemologies and methodologies), and the range of solutions to health problems that are seen to be viable and are even on one's radar.

Significantly, these different perspectives may be separate, but they are certainly not equal in visibility or prominence. As articulated in their still highly relevant book, Tesh (1988) argues that different theories of disease causation (Tesh offered germ, lifestyle, and environmental as key 20th-century theories) have "hidden arguments" (from the book's title) reflecting the political and ideological implications of those causes and corresponding prevention policy. Those hidden arguments also explain why some explanations rise to prominence over others. Those focusing on biomedical or behavioural factors become dominant because they align with powerful capitalist interests, such as medical, pharmaceutical, and wellness industries in which solutions of an individualized and technical nature are highly profitable, regardless of 'effectiveness' (itself a contentious notion). This dominance of reductive, individualized perspectives is enhanced by a carefully constructed veil of scientific objectivity and neutrality, which has immense epistemic power (Valles 2018; see also Chapter 2 in this volume).

As long recognized by critical scholars, the hegemonic 'common sense' narrative of biomedical and behavioural perspectives serves to obscure the structural nature of causes that are embedded in our economic and political systems (see also Chapter 4 in this volume). Doing so ensures that those systems and structures are not seriously considered as foci for improving well-being and health equity. This, in turn, achieves the entirely intended effect of maintaining capitalism's status quo and serving the interests of its beneficiaries – political and economic elites. These dynamics, illuminated by a political economy lens, play out importantly across the knowledge production process, including research agenda setting and funding, and scholarly publishing.

Research agendas and funding

Dominant, reductive perspectives on health powerfully shape processes of research agenda setting and funding. They do so by setting contours and limits – which may be explicit but are usually implicit ('hidden', as per Tesh's [1988] thesis) – around what is deemed important or legitimate to study.

Examples from Canada are illustrative. Bungay et al. (2023) critically analysed the nature of funding for sex work-related health research in Canada. This work was anchored in the public and global health imperative of supporting the health and human rights of adults engaged in sex work and the need for an evidentiary foundation for such support. Based on the argument that research funding allocation taps into the complex social processes that are inherent to the logic and strategy of building an evidence base for health improvement, Bungay et al. (2023) examined the scope, focus, and extent of operating grants awarded by the federal health research funding agency, the Canadian Institutes of Health Research (CIHR), between 2003 and 2010. Grounded in critical perspectives on occupational stigma, the authors were specifically interested in whether and how the research funding patterns contributed to, or challenged, normative assumptions about sex work and thus health inequities.

Bungay et al. (2023) showed that the funded research tended to problematize sex workers' health in a certain way, namely as situated in a street marketplace context focusing on HIV and sexually transmitted infections. Research questions were found to emphasize behaviours of sex workers such as condom use or drug use. There was less attention to the socio-structural context of sex work, including racism, classism, and sexism, and how those play out in sex workers' lives and livelihoods. The authors also found that the applicants were tightly networked, with the 64 grants being held by 48 people, 18 of whom held principal or co-principal applicant roles on multiple grants. Collectively, the authors argue these findings shed light on how the processes and dynamics shaping what research is funded can perpetuate both stigmatizing narratives about sex work and imbalances in what is studied and from what perspective(s). Moreover, to the extent that research shapes practice and policy designed to support the health and well-being of sex workers, the authors point out that a narrow focus in funded research can serve to obscure the need for socio-structural policy and programming such as that which centres harm reduction, poverty reduction, and gender-based violence (Bungay et al. 2023).

In another example from the Canadian context, Medvedyuk et al. (2018) critically analysed how the relationship between obesity and health was represented in agenda-setting documents, including public health reports and clinical practice guidelines. 'Obesity', it must be tangentially noted, is a focus of rich critical scholarship in public health and fat studies literatures where it has been very effectively problematized (see, e.g., Bombak et al. 2022; McNaughton 2011; Monaghan et al. 2018).

Situated within those scholarly literatures, Medvedyuk et al. (2018) first outlined five different models of how the relationship between obesity and health can be understood. For example, one model, highly dominant, is that obesity itself causes poor health outcomes; in other words, obesity, which is seen to result from one's behavioural choices, causes health problems through physiological effects. A second model holds that obesity, shaped by social determinants such as low income, insecure employment, and food and housing insecurity, causes adverse health outcomes. While this second model recognizes the role of social factors in shaping eating and exercise patterns, its failure to question the link between obesity and health means that it often manifests in a downstream manner, such as focusing on behaviours of persons living in disadvantaged social circumstances. A third model (Model 4 in the paper) is that obesity, shaped by social determinants, does not contribute to adverse health outcomes. Anchored in critical perspectives, this latter model directs attention to social determinants of health (SDH) and minimizes or denies a role for obesity itself in producing health problems. It emphasizes that a preoccupation with obesity (as per the first two models above) persists not because of scientific evidence of harms but rather – as per a political economy perspective – because of its alignment with powerful interests. These include strong and long-standing societal discourse around ideal bodies and vilification of fat, which underpin a highly lucrative weight-loss industry (Medvedyuk et al. 2018).

Focusing on Canadian public health reports produced by organizations, such as the Public Health Agency of Canada, the Canadian Institute for Health Information, and Public Health Ontario, Medvedyuk et al. (2018) showed, firstly, that these agenda-setting documents embraced alarmist language around obesity, portraying it as a serious public health threat requiring urgent action. Although various factors were acknowledged in these documents as contributing to obesity, they ultimately positioned obesity as stemming primarily from poor lifestyle and behavioural habits, for which individually based and downstream settings-based interventions were seen as suitable approaches to prevention, thus aligning with Models 1 and 2 above. The authors effectively argued that, to the extent that these narratives support calls for funding for biomedical and behaviourally oriented obesity research, they perpetuate a downstream narrative that leaves root causes of poor health untouched and intact. These include the power of industries that profit from demonizing obesity and the neoliberal political economic structures (e.g. weak regulatory policy) that support them (Medvedyuk et al. 2018). A recent and highly problematic version of this reductive orientation is personalized and *precision* health and medicine; see Chapter 3 in this volume.

It is important to emphasize the nuance of such critical work. Even within mainstream perspectives, it is not hard to accept that social factors could be relevant. Indeed, agenda-setting documents in public health nearly always mention social factors. As Raphael (2011; see also Raphael and Bryant 2023) notes, the idea of upstream social determinants has achieved a prominence that makes it difficult for policymakers, health researchers, and professionals to ignore altogether (see also Chapter 4 in this volume). The insidiousness of the biomedical/behavioural hegemony is that one can acknowledge the role of upstream factors but still land, in a seemingly logical manner, on a particular behaviour, risk factor, or disease, conceptualized in a downstream, individualized manner, as the main problem and focus for knowledge production and mobilization.

The global political economic context of knowledge production

Critical scholarship has shed important light on political economic dynamics shaping public health agenda setting globally. An important paper by Storeng et al. (2016), for example, considered the 'rise from obscurity' of a particular metric – the *maternal mortality ratio* (MMR) – to become a major global health indicator, despite significant concerns by experts about the metric's reliability. Storeng et al.'s (2016) work is situated in the neoliberal political economic context, including its assumptions that healthcare priorities should be shaped by cost-effectiveness logics and business management models and achieved through market-driven approaches and public–private partnerships, under the dominant leadership of business-oriented institutions like the Gates Foundation. In such a context, the authors argue, *metrics*, including MMR, become central to solving complex global health challenges.

Based on interviews with international academic researchers and measurement experts (e.g. epidemiologists and demographers) in Europe and North America, Storeng et al. (2016) identified important tensions experienced by those experts over the use of the MMR as a key global health indicator. On the one hand, experts recognized that a focus on metrics was important in that it underpinned commitments to transparency and accountability and allowed for better understanding of 'what works' to address maternal health. At the same time, experts identified a more complex set of factors, including a perceived need to respond to donors' (such as the Gates Foundation) demand for data to justify investment flows and to produce data that would allow maternal health to remain a global-level political priority in an increasingly competitive policy space (Storeng et al. 2016). In the context of these political economic dynamics, the MMR's 'rise from obscurity' to a prominent indicator of progress towards global development goals (e.g. the Sustainable Development Goals (SDGs)) served, according to the authors, to divert attention *away* from other important activities, like efforts to strengthen data monitoring and health system infrastructure at national and sub-national levels. Storeng et al. (2016) conclude that the emphasis on the MMR resembles what anthropologist Vincanne Adams called "micropractices of neoliberalism" – practices that "are not necessarily designed with neoliberal outcomes in mind, but they work seamlessly with the political aspirations of neoliberal reforms" (p. 164) and thus serve to undermine community health.

Notwithstanding the increasing global power of neoliberal institutions like the World Bank and the Gates Foundation, an analysis of the global political economy of knowledge production must also examine intergovernmental organizations, perhaps most notably the World Health Organization (WHO), which itself is shaped by broader neoliberal dynamics. A recent contribution by Lee (2023) considered the political economic factors shaping WHO agenda setting, by examining "the politics of ignorance" (from the article's title) in the context of WHO debates over health inequities experienced by sexual and gender minority populations (SGM).

Lee (2023) specifically aimed to explain a decision by the WHO Executive Board between 2013 and 2016 to "suspend and eventually end the discussion over

SGM health" (p. 48) or, in other words, to do nothing about SGM health. This decision (to do nothing) was despite, and contrary to, the WHO's legal obligation to promote knowledge generation that aims to tackle barriers to everyone achieving high levels of health. To shed light on the significant, but largely invisible, processes underlying the WHO's decision to do nothing, Lee's (2023) work was theoretically anchored in the *sociology of nothing* and the *sociology of ignorance*, which argue that "nothing, just like anything, has a traceable social life" (p. 49). Understanding and explaining *nothing* thus involve considering 'unmarked' events and experiences, as well as things that never happened, for example, data collection activities that were *not* requested by the WHO.

Employing a poststructuralist approach, Lee (2023) set out to 'redo' the relevant WHO documents (i.e. meeting records, regional offices' documents, other WHO publications) in a way that "bring[s] the omitted – the once there but has now disappeared – back into sight" (p. 50). Concretely, this involved paying attention to dominant discourses and how they are affirmed and depoliticized, as well as to items that were bracketed, footnoted, and deleted. Collectively, this approach allowed for the identification of contradictions between actors mobilizing the discourse of evidence-based public health around SGM health.

On the surface, the WHO's decision to do nothing around SGM health was based on a lack of evidence. However, rather than prompting WHO action (as per its legal obligation), the lack of evidence was used as a rationale for intentionally neglecting the health concerns of particular social groups. Lee (2023) identified that this manifested as two forms of 'non-evidence'. First is *non-recognition*; this is an act of omission of certain SGMs from the discourse, for example, street cruising men who have sex with men. The second is *mis-recognition*, which in this case was the neglect of SGM health issues that were not related to sexually transmitted infections. Mis-recognition, the authors argue, stems from social exclusion due to monosexual assumptions. Both forms of non-evidence served to further silence SGM's on the global health policy agenda. Lee's (2023) work thus sheds light on structural political economic factors that significantly shape research agenda setting by this important intergovernmental organization.

Scholarly journals and the publishing landscape

In addition to research agendas and funding priorities, political and economic factors strongly shape scholarly publishing. Indeed, it would be highly remiss not to critically situate any discussion of academic publishing within the contemporary publishing landscape. This landscape is characterized by corporate domination and the commodification of knowledge, which has led to a massive increase in the volume of material being published as well as the resulting strain on peer-review processes (Bell and Green 2020; Green and Speed 2018). As per a political economy framework, this landscape can be understood in terms of conflict between actors with competing interests – in this case, the profit imperative of corporate publishing on the one hand and the knowledge generation and publication imperative of academic researchers on the other. This conflict plays out within a political economic context that privileges some groups and perspectives – based on approaches, professions, and positionality, for example, over others.

For scholars starting out today, aspects of the contemporary publishing landscape, such as the very large number of journals and published papers, the impossibly short turnaround times for manuscript review and revisions, and the ubiquity of high article processing fees, may be quite familiar. In fact, this is a relatively recent phenomenon. Bell et al. (2021) describe how the late 1990s was a period of rapid corporate consolidation in scholarly publishing. The experience of the journal *Critical Public Health* is instructive (see also the Introduction chapter of this volume). Following its origins as an informal pamphlet called *Radical Community Medicine*, which was founded by a critically oriented collective, in 1998 it became a fully refereed international journal owned and distributed by the academic publisher Carfax. However, as Bell et al. (2021, p. 377) describe, "the ink was barely dry" on this arrangement before Carfax was bought out by Routledge, which was in turn bought out by the Taylor & Francis Group, which merged with Informa in 2004.

Such rapid and large-scale changes in journal ownership and distribution were common: citing Larivière et al. (2015), Bell et al. (2021) note that by 2015, 70% of all social science publications indexed in Web of Science were published by five corporate publishers: Elsevier, Springer, Taylor & Francis, Wiley-Blackwell, and Sage. This corporate monopolization permitted an arrangement where higher and lower prestige journals were 'bundled' together in profit-generating subscription packages for university libraries. Together with author-pays (fee-for-publication) models of open access, this has yielded massive profits (reflecting massive profit margins) for the big publishers while simultaneously – and fundamentally – reshaping the scholarly publishing landscape. The reshaping is far from innocuous and demands critical analysis. A political economy analysis illuminates that the relationship between the owners of the means of scholarly publication (the corporate publishers) and the 'workers' (i.e. academic authors, reviewers, and editors, for whom this work is inherent to their jobs) has become one of exploitation, where academic labour is the key mechanism for-profit generation. This is compounded by the private extraction by corporate publishers of public capital in the form of publicly funded research – that is, scholarly research that is largely funded by national and sub-national governments. Indeed, there are important questions to be asked about who pays, and who benefits, from this arrangement.

These trends, while affecting scholarly publishing across the board, have particular implications for critically oriented scholarship which is centrally concerned with issues of equity and power. Certainly, the fee-for-publication model exacerbates inequities based on material resources (who has the money to pay), but it goes much deeper than that. Critical scholarship by its nature goes against the grain of mainstream research agendas and funding priorities. It is thus frequently done 'off the side of one's desk', either on the periphery of a funded project or unfunded altogether. This is perhaps particularly true for early career scholars and independent researchers, who lack the security of tenured academics. By further limiting publication opportunities for critical scholarship, article processing charges (APCs) have the effect of further silencing critical voices and strengthening already dominant ones. Indeed, from the perspective of critical scholarship as "an *intellectual project* driven by a concern about the power relations of knowledge production – especially the role of corporate influences, north–south inequalities, and the politics of disciplinarity" (p. 378, emphasis in original), one could argue without exaggeration that the contemporary publishing model is simply incompatible with critical scholarship in public health and other fields, and the experience with *Critical Public Health* and its owner/publisher Taylor & Francis is illustrative (Bell et al. 2021).

Political economy of scholarly publishing and global inequalities

These political economic dynamics have global implications in the form of north–south inequalities in scholarly publishing. The existence and persistence of such inequalities are well established. For example, based on a descriptive analysis of articles published in highly ranked public health journals in 2016, Plancikova et al. (2021) identified that over 80% were conducted in high-income countries and 84% of authors were based in high-income countries. The 'open science movement', with its aim of making scientific research and its dissemination available to everyone, came with the promise of redressing this significant imbalance. However, within the contemporary, highly corporatized scholarly publishing landscape and the broader economic context of neoliberal capitalism, this is not how it has played out.

A study by Bezuidenhout et al. (2017) sheds light on the promises of open science and some factors that obstruct the realization of the ambitious vision. These authors applied Sen's capabilities approach and, in particular, Sen's concept of 'conversion factors' to consider not only the *presence* of online data but also challenges to its productive *use*. Based on the experiences of Kenyan and South African researchers, the authors identified numerous challenges to making use of 'freely available' data. One is financial barriers, such as membership fees required for data sharing. A second challenge concerns employment-related demands and constraints that result in researchers accessing journals at home on personal time, which may be complicated by unreliable infrastructure and/or prohibitive cost. A final challenge, also related to infrastructure, relates to the need to purchase software and hardware out of pocket. These findings show that, to the extent that the open science movement is reduced to making data and research 'freely available', it obscures significant challenges to global publishing equity that are fundamentally anchored in global social and economic inequities. Bezuidenhout et al. (2017) effectively argue that "The promises of Open Science imply a set of expectations about what different publics hope to gain from research, how accountability and participation can be enhanced, and what makes science public in the first place" (p. 39). Their work makes clear that those expectations must be analysed critically.

Although cost-related barriers to knowledge production, such as article processing fees, are very important, north–south inequalities in publishing are far deeper and more complicated than that. Beyond useful or interesting ideas or findings, publishing in established journals requires an ability to navigate publishing cultures. This includes academic writing skills and the ability to effectively select and tailor one's work to journals. It also requires 'stylistic capital', meaning the ability to effectively craft arguments for largely anglophone scholarly communities (Allman 2019; Green and Speed 2018). This complexity is obscured by corporate publishers' highly inadequate 'solutions' to north–south inequities, such as open-access fee subsidies for authors in lower-income countries.

The complexity of the dynamics at play in global knowledge production is put into stark relief in the context of so-called predatory publishing, a phenomenon that has accompanied the broader commodification and corporatization of scholarly publishing. 'Predatory' journals and publishers are loosely defined as those that are questionable in terms of quality and credibility due to practices such as minimal or no peer review and apparent willingness to publish work of low quality or importance so long as the author is willing to pay the open-access fee (Beall n.d.). Critical scholarship has contributed importantly to problematizing the 'predatory' discourse. Allman (2019), for example, has emphasized that the line separating legitimate or credible publishing on the one hand, from 'pseudo' (including predatory) publishing on the other, is 'porous'. This is no surprise to any author who has tried to discern whether a particular journal is 'predatory' or not.

Moreover, and more importantly, Allman (2019) argues that the 'porous' division between credible and pseudo tends to align – explicitly or implicitly – with the division between more and less developed parts of the world. Using a creative approach of *case story methodology*, Allman (2019) illustrates these divisions by constructing a narrative of a publisher of scholarly content that could – superficially – be seen as 'predatory'. The analysis is guided by the interesting concept of 'social banditry', where the activities of groups of people living on the margins of society are considered criminal by those in power, but empowering or emancipative by the groups themselves. From this perspective, Allman (2019) effectively demonstrates how so-called predatory journals and practices can instead be seen as a form of production, often originating in the global south, that seeks to access resources from the overprivileged global north, thus benefiting the well-being of its communities. These insights are significant with respect to deepening understanding of global knowledge production inequities and for reframing the 'predatory' publication discourse.

Scholarly publishing in the post-truth era

Green and Speed (2018) situate 'predatory' publishing within the so-called post-truth context. 'Post-truth', for these authors, refers to political and popular discourse where objective facts are less influential in shaping public opinion than appeals to emotion or personal belief (Speed and Mannion 2017). In this context, Green and Speed (2018) remark on the considerable momentum that has accumulated around defending academic publishing standards. They first acknowledge that there are, indeed, important reasons to focus on defending academic publishing standards. For example, one consequence of the commodification of knowledge is that it has incentivized researchers to 'salami slice' their work. This results in massive numbers of publications that are excessively incremental or trivial. Moreover, the volume of incremental work tends to perpetuate dominant reductive and individualized ways of thinking about health, as noted above, because such work is more easily funded and is quicker to complete and publish (Haines-Saah and McLaren 2023).

However, Green and Speed (2018) argue that the 'defence of science' reaction to the 'predatory' trend represents an oversimplification and demands a critical gaze. Consistent with Allman's (2019) work, Green and Speed (2018) argue that the predatory framing obscures and thus perpetuates underlying global inequities of power, in their words: "[d]enigrating emerging forms of publishing to defend 'standards' in traditional outlets can be seen … as a form of cultural imperialism" (p. 130). Their arguments demonstrate the importance of asking questions like who is making claims about 'predatory' practices and to what end. Indeed, there is considerable irony when labels of 'predatory' apply disproportionately to journals *outside of* the 'big five' corporate publishers, when those publishers strongly shape what is seen as credible in high-income countries.

Layered on top of these political economic dynamics of the contemporary publishing landscape, and magnifying many of its problems, came the COVID-19 pandemic. During 2020 – the first year of expansive measures including lockdown in much of the world – journal editors commiserated over the massive increase in the number of submissions. This was coupled with what felt like an equally large increase in difficulty securing reviewers. Assurances from corporate publishers like Taylor & Francis that they would "prioritiz[e] rapid publication of COVID-19 materials" (Bell and Green 2020, p. 380) were disjointed from the experiences and workload of editors and reviewers. This was especially true for critically oriented journals, which served to further cement the positioning of such journals – from the publisher's point of view – as commodities that were somehow separate from the (largely unpaid) intellectual community that produces them (Bell et al. 2021).

As discussed by Bell and Green (2020), the 'agility' of scientific publishing during the pandemic was viewed positively by some, especially in comparison with the more typical (pre-pandemic) pace of scientific communication. Importantly, however, there was also some uneasiness about the speed at which research was being produced and made available, often as pre-prints (work that has not yet been through peer review). Although pre-prints are usually labelled, thus in principle allowing readers to interpret the content with that draft status in mind, the rapid emergence of pre-prints in the pandemic context inevitably increased the potential for work that was weak, misleading, or even wrong, to be shared and amplified.

Moreover, as an illustration of the important contribution of critical scholarship in this space, Bell and Green (2020) point out that these pandemic-related trends in publishing have strong potential to exacerbate existing inequities in knowledge production. This will require further study as more time has passed, but one example is gender inequalities in publishing, stemming from highly gendered impacts of the pandemic, such as disruptions to school and childcare, the brunt of which largely fell to women and mothers. Another example is global north–south inequities. At *Critical Public Health*, for example, the pandemic brought with it an avalanche of submissions, many of which were out of scope, of which many came from parts of the world that are less well represented in the journal (and in established scholarly journals in general) in the first place.

Conclusion

Critical perspectives in public health are committed to rigorously surfacing and challenging the dynamics of power that cause certain perspectives, topics, and approaches to achieve dominance, while others are marginalized or omitted altogether. In contrast to hegemonic narratives underpinned by intersecting bio-medical/behavioural approaches to health and neoliberal political economy, what becomes dominant is in no way 'natural' or neutral. Illuminating the usually hidden processes that make it seem that way is an important goal of critical scholarship in public health, including the dynamics of knowledge production.

As articulated in the first edition of this volume by Green and Labonté (2008), the process of illumination can take the form of a critical voice *for* public health and a critique *of* public health (see also the Introduction chapter). A critical voice *for* public health means a stance for uncovering the health-damaging effects of particular social structures in their political and historical contexts and challenging those structures. A critique *of* public health includes looking inward to ask diffi-cult questions about our field and to constantly question our own taken-for-granted assumptions. In this chapter, we have attempted to illustrate how both outward- and inward-looking approaches, anchored in a political economy framework, can shed important light on forms of power and conflict as they play out in knowledge pro-duction. from research agenda setting to research funding to scholarly publishing. These dynamics also, of course, strongly shape which knowledge is mobilized, how, and to what end(s).

A political economy of health framework foregrounds inequities of resources and power towards understanding how poor health and health inequities are generated and experienced. Importantly, the framework also provides insights into ways forward. In its Marxist tradition, political economy centres on competing interests and conflict between class groups – originally between owners of cap-ital and the working class. Just as conflict between these groups produces harms to workers, so too has conflict historically produced improvements – via worker organizing and mobilization – to such determinants of health as income, benefits, occupational safety, and legal protections (Chernomas and Hudson 2013; Finkel 2012). The Marxist frame has, in the 20th century, been elaborated to recognize nuance across classes and the imperative of power analysis across intersecting dimensions of gender, race, ethnicity, etc. (Grabb 2007; Harvey 2021).

This frame raises at least three key ideas for rebalancing power within the political economy of knowledge production. Starting with scholarly publishing, one important idea is to pursue alternatives to the current model of corporate publishing (see also the Introduction chapter in this volume). Important work by Bell et al. (2021) discusses so-called diamond open-access models of publishing, which are based on an economically viable cost-recovery approach, rather than a profit-generating approach, thus disrupting a key element of capitalism. The diamond model permits the publication to be free to the end user and with no charges to the submitting author. Encouragingly, this model is gaining momentum, especially in the social sciences and humanities. One example is the Open Library of Humanities, which is an open-access publisher of internationally leading academic scholarship in the humanities whose goal is "to liberate university research from community control" based on the belief that "scholarship should be academic-led and community-owned".[1]

Pursuing alternatives to dominant corporate publishing models requires a strong base of support that, similar to advances gained by organized activism in labour and civil rights communities, is positioned and poised to mobilize. The second idea thus concerns the need to build and sustain robust scholarly communities for critical public health. One example is the evolving Critical Public Health Network.[2] This is a virtual international community that aims to (1) act as an advocate for the critical public health scholarly community; (2) offer a point of contact for those interested in the intersection of social science/humanities and public health; and (3) provide a network for information/knowledge exchange amongst members.

The third idea is that to sustain a critical public health movement towards an alternative political economic paradigm, including for knowledge production, an incoming base of scholars, practitioners, and activists who are capable of thinking critically and structurally is required. This imperative draws one's attention to our education systems producing the next generation of public health workers (where 'workers' includes researchers, scholars, and practitioners). Within the increasingly corporatized landscape of post-secondary education, important scholarship has identified that critical perspectives in public health education programmes – including critical social theories and non-dominant methodologies – are absent or relegated to the periphery (Harvey and McGladrey 2019; Skinner 2019; Yassi et al. 2019). If we wish to sustain robust public health communities that are equipped to notice and call out when certain perspectives are rising to the top while others are sidelined, the highly institutionalized inequities embedded in mainstream public health education must be redressed.

Notes

1 Available at: www.openlibhums.org.
2 Available at: www.cphn.net.

References

Allman, D. (2019) 'Pseudo or perish: problematizing the "predatory" in global health publishing', *Critical Public Health*, 29(4), pp. 413–423. Available at: https://doi.org/10.1080/09581596.2019.1606417.
Beall, J. (no date) 'Beall's list (archived version)'. Available at: https://beallslist.net.
Bell, K. and Green, J. (2020) 'Premature evaluation? Some cautionary thoughts on global pandemics and scholarly publishing', *Critical Public Health*, 30(4), pp. 379–383. Available at: https://doi.org/10.1080/09581596.2020.1769406.

Bell, K. *et al.* (2021) '"Open" relationships: reflections on the role of the journal in the contemporary scholarly publishing landscape', *Critical Public Health*, 31(4), pp. 377–380. Available at: https://doi.org/10.1080/09581596.2021.1958512.

Bezuidenhout, L. *et al.* (2017) ' "$100 is not much to you": open science and neglected accessibilities for scientific research in Africa', *Critical Public Health*, 27(1), pp. 39–49. Available at: https://doi.org/10.1080/09581596.2016.1252832.

Bombak, A.E., Adams, L. and Thille, P. (2022) 'Drivers of medicalization in the Canadian Adult Obesity Clinical Practice Guidelines', *Canadian Journal of Public Health*, 113(5), pp. 743–748. Available at: https://doi.org/10.17269/s41997-022-00662-4.

Bungay, V. *et al.* (2023) 'Gaps in health research related to sex work: an analysis of Canadian health research funding', *Critical Public Health*, 33(1), pp. 72–82. Available at: https://doi.org/10.1080/09581596.2021.1987385.

Chernomas, R. and Hudson, I. (2013) *To live and die in America: class, power, health, and healthcare*. London: Pluto Press [u.a.] (The future of world capitalism).

Davidson, A. (2019) *Social determinants of health: a comparative approach*. Second edition. Don Mills, Ontario, Canada: Oxford University Press.

Finkel, A. (ed.) (2012) *Working people in Alberta: a history*. Edmonton: AU Press (Working Canadians, books from the CCLH).

Grabb, E.G. (2007) *Theories of social inequality*. 5th ed. Toronto, ON: Thomson/Nelson.

Green, J. and Labonté, R. (eds.) (2008) *Critical perspectives in public health*. London: Routledge.

Green, J. and Speed, E. (2018) 'Critical analysis, credibility, and the politics of publishing in an era of "fake news" ', *Critical Public Health*, 28(2), pp. 129–131. Available at: https://doi.org/10.1080/09581596.2017.1421597.

Haines-Saah, R. and McLaren, L. (2023) 'A cautionary tale: university institutes of public health must "walk the talk" ', *Canadian Journal of Public Health*, 114(5), pp. 710–713. Available at: https://doi.org/10.17269/s41997-023-00815-z.

Harvey, M. (2021) 'The political economy of health: revisiting its Marxian origins to address 21st-century health inequalities', *American Journal of Public Health*, 111(2), pp. 293–300. Available at: https://doi.org/10.2105/AJPH.2020.305996.

Harvey, M. and McGladrey, M. (2019) 'Explaining the origins and distribution of health and disease: an analysis of epidemiologic theory in core Master of Public Health coursework in the United States', *Critical Public Health*, 29(1), pp. 5–17. Available at: https://doi.org/10.1080/09581596.2018.1535698.

Labonté, R. and Stuckler, D. (2016) 'The rise of neoliberalism: how bad economics imperils health and what to do about it', *Journal of Epidemiology and Community Health*, 70(3), pp. 312–318. Available at: https://doi.org/10.1136/jech-2015-206295.

Larivière, V., Haustein, S. and Mongeon, P. (2015) 'The oligopoly of academic publishers in the digital era', *PLOS One*, 10(6), p. e0127502. Available at: https://doi.org/10.1371

Lee, P.-H. (2023) 'Un(ac)countable no-bodies: the politics of ignorance in global health policymaking', *Critical Public Health*, 33(1), pp. 48–59. Available at: https://doi.org/10.1080/09581596.2022.2025578.

McNaughton, D. (2011) 'From the womb to the tomb: obesity and maternal responsibility', *Critical Public Health*, 21(2), pp. 179–190. Available at: https://doi.org/10.1080/09581596.2010.523680.

Medvedyuk, S., Ali, A. and Raphael, D. (2018) 'Ideology, obesity and the social determinants of health: a critical analysis of the obesity and health relationship', *Critical Public Health*, 28(5), pp. 573–585. Available at: https://doi.org/10.1080/09581596.2017.1356910.

Monaghan, L.F., Bombak, A.E. and Rich, E. (2018) 'Obesity, neoliberalism and epidemic psychology: critical commentary and alternative approaches to public health', *Critical Public Health*, 28(5), pp. 498–508. Available at: https://doi.org/10.1080/09581 596.2017.1371278.

Plancikova, D., Duric, P. and O'May, F. (2021) 'High-income countries remain overrepresented in highly ranked public health journals: a descriptive analysis of research settings and authorship affiliations', *Critical Public Health*, 31(4), pp. 487–493. Available at: https://doi.org/10.1080/09581596.2020.1722313.

Raphael, D. (2011) 'A discourse analysis of the social determinants of health', *Critical Public Health*, 21(2), pp. 221–236. Available at: https://doi.org/10.1080/09581596.2010.485606.

Raphael, D. and Bryant, T. (2023) 'Socialism as the way forward: updating a discourse analysis of the social determinants of health', *Critical Public Health*, 33(4), pp. 387–394. Available at: https://doi.org/10.1080/09581596.2023.2178387.

Skinner, D. (2019) 'Challenges in public health pedagogy', *Critical Public Health*, 29(1), pp. 1–4. Available at: https://doi.org/10.1080/09581596.2019.1538078.

Speed, E. and Mannion, R. (2017) 'The rise of post-truth populism in pluralist liberal democracies: challenges for health policy', *International Journal of Health Policy and Management*, 6(5), pp. 249–251. Available at: https://doi.org/10.15171/ijhpm.2017.19.

Storeng, K.T. and Béhague, D.P. (2016) '"Guilty until proven innocent": the contested use of maternal mortality indicators in global health', *Critical Public Health*, 27(2), pp. 163–176. Available at: https://doi.org/10.1080/09581596.2016.1259459.

Tesh, S.N. (1988) *Hidden arguments: political ideology and disease prevention policy.* New Brunswick, N.J.: Rutgers University Press.

Valles, S.A. (2018) *Philosophy of population health: philosophy for a new public health era.* London: Routledge.

Yassi, A. *et al.* (2019) 'Is public health training in Canada meeting current needs? Defrosting the paradigm freeze to respond to the post-truth era', *Critical Public Health*, 29(1), pp. 40–47. Available at: https://doi.org/10.1080/09581596.2017.1384796.

2 Making evidence

Complexity, trials, and epistemic justice

Over the last two decades, the utility of the conventional 'toolbox' of public health methods, rooted largely in ever more sophisticated statistical analyses of epidemiological data and in evaluative approaches based on experimental trial logics, has come under increasing pressure. This has been driven in part by the pragmatic limitations of this toolbox for addressing pressing questions for public health policy and practice, particularly around building an evidence base for what works in addressing upstream determinants of health and health equity. However, more fundamentally, limitations arise from a range of epistemic injustices. Evidence is systematically excluded at the micro-level, by the methods we use, as well as at the macro-level of the political economy of knowledge production discussed in Chapter 1 of this volume.

The so-called complexity turn (Urry 2005) has framed much recent critical literature on public health methods, with a search for designs and approaches that can adequately account for the complex ways in which health is sustained or damaged and which can make useful evaluative evidence. This has reoriented public health methodology towards various kinds of system thinking, with interventions framed as 'disruptions in systems' (Hawe et al. 2009). One outcome has been an overdue reappraisal of the randomized controlled trial (RCT) as a privileged source of evidence given its limitations in addressing causation in complex systems. To an extent, the COVID-19 pandemic has been an accelerant for these critiques. As Greenhalgh (2020) noted:

> Population-wide public health efforts are typically iterative, locally-grown and path-dependent, and they have an established methodology for rapid evaluation and adaptation … But evidence-based medicine has tended to classify such designs as 'low methodological quality' … . Whilst this has been recognised as a problem in public health practice for some time … the inadequacy of the dominant paradigm has suddenly become mission-critical.
>
> (p. 1)

In times of crisis, public health science plays out in public and in real time. Responses to the COVID-19 pandemic, in many jurisdictions, generated unparalleled levels of

DOI: 10.4324/9781003654650-3

citizen engagement with, and critique of, public health research, as techniques such as mathematical modelling moved to centre stage in the public arena (Rhodes et al. 2020) and became topics of everyday debate (Green et al. 2022). As Greenhalgh (2020) argued, rapidly implemented trials were vital for producing information around issues such as vaccine effectiveness. Yet, many of the questions that became pressing during the pandemic – around the sustainability of interventions to change social behaviours or the best ways to ensure public information was disseminated – required what she called "epistemology and methods to study how best to cope with uncertainty, unpredictability and non-linear causality" (p. 2). This presents challenges that are both technical (e.g., how to integrate a greater range of causal logics or how to design studies that provide useful and relevant knowledge for policy actors) and political. Methodological norms – what counts as 'robust' evidence – can systematically exclude some kinds of evidence (Indigenous knowledge, experiential knowledge), and they can have looping effects that reproduce the very inequalities they aim to study, such as reifying health-related identities.

This chapter reviews the contributions of critical public health scholars to addressing these challenges, from early critiques of the evidence-based medicine (EBM) movement through efforts to 'tinker with trials' to develop more fitting methodologies for a complex world, and in turn to critiques of simplistic calls for a 'complexity turn' in public health as a solution. Without embedding methodological development in a broader political programme of epistemic justice, such solutions will inevitably be partial.

Assembling knowledge: the problematic nature of the public health evidence base

From its origins in the early 1990s, EBM expanded rapidly as an approach advocated for not only clinical decisions, but also, increasingly, health and social policy decisions (Mykhalovskiy and Weir 2004; Pearce and Raman 2014). The successes of EBM in both the clinic (Pope 2003) and the public health front line (Owusu-Addo et al. 2017) may have been partial. The forms EBM takes on the ground are certainly diverse and context specific, as Borozdina (2023) documents in the context of contemporary Russian health care. Certainly, in many of the fields in which public health policy is made, formal assessments of research evidence may be a minor strand of decision-making in practice (Phillips and Green 2015; Stevens 2011). However, if claims about the hegemony of EBM may be overblown, arguably, a rhetorical adherence to the principles that decisions *should* be made in the light of the 'best' evidence is now difficult to resist.

The rise of EBM has been attributed variously to neoliberal drivers such as needs for standardization, technologies of managerial control over medicine, and cost constraints – although, as Mykhalovskiy and Weir (2004) noted, these outcomes neither necessarily flow from the application of EBM in clinical settings, nor do they inherently align to its founding principles. Rather than accounting for the ways in which EBM does or doesn't get adopted, or how it conflicts with more humanistic forms of medical care, Mykhalovskiy and Weir suggested the driving questions for critical scholars should be empirical ones: around how different logics of medicine coexist and what underpinning assumptions contribute to making up the evidence base. These questions have been taken up over the last 15 years, with critical scholars unpacking the various ways in which EBM (as both a project and a practice) intersects with public health research, as well as the policies and programmes built on that research evidence.

One instructive example is Bell's (2012) analysis of the 'creep' of EBM into fields of public health through a detailed analysis of the Cochrane Collaboration's systematic review of physician advice to give up smoking. She notes the elision of social context in the reviews of trials: the genders, social relations, and structural constraints of trial participants are rendered invisible; different time periods (with very different smoking policy environments) are combined; and effects are averaged out across countries with very different legislative settings. While subgroup analysis can address these issues to an extent, Bell's point is that there is an underlying assumption in the methodologies around the stability of 'human behaviour' and universal psychological mechanisms, as if they were separate from the contexts in which they are actualized. The 'creep' of methodologies from clinical medicine renders both behavioural interventions and human responses as discrete and as belonging to individuals: capable of being researched in the same way as medications in physiological bodies.

An over-reliance on conventional evidence hierarchies to inform 'the evidence base' has long been recognized as particularly problematic for many questions in public health. This is, to be sure, also a challenge for clinical medicine, which also struggles with the diverse kinds of evidence (Wieringa et al. 2021) and 'non-knowledge' (Knaapen 2013) that need to be incorporated into clinical guidelines. For public health questions, though, there is perhaps a larger hinterland of 'unknowns'. That is, there is a paucity of evidence deriving from RCTs on interventions at the upstream, structural level, and an overproduction of evidence pertaining to downstream, individualistic and behavioural interventions. Indeed, to apply the methods of the trial – designed to look at effects in individual patients – to the population is what Davey-Smith and Ebrahim (2001) called a 'category error'. If the strongest evidence is considered that from trials, then the available evidence is likely to be largely on relatively low-level factors and technological interventions, rather than the upstream determinants that will (theoretically) have more impact on health. On smoking, then, as Bell (2012) demonstrated, we have far more evidence on individual behavioural interventions than we do on social or environmental interventions, as the former are more likely to have been subject to RCT evaluation (Bell 2012). Similar limitations have been documented across many other public health domains. On transport systems, for instance, Ogilvie et al. (2005) conducted a systematic review of interventions that supported a shift from car travel to active transport, noting a similar imbalance in available evidence. They suggested that an 'inverse evidence law' operated: evidence that is most needed (on structural interventions) was least likely to exist. Thus, if systematic reviews focus on trial evidence, they are less likely to include evidence for social or environmental interventions that might have a larger impact on transport mode shifts in healthier directions.

The inappropriateness of RCT methods for addressing the outcomes of complex interventions in complex systems (i.e. most of the issues faced by public health) has led to a growing interest in quasi-experimental methods. So-called natural experiments – events not within the control of the researcher – have been hailed as ripe for evaluations and as potentially filling the gap for public health policy and practice (Craig et al. 2022; Craig et al. 2025). Since the 2010s, there has been a marked increase in the number of 'natural experiments' appearing in public and environmental health (Herrick and Bell 2024), evaluating interventions such as new laws or policies. However, many of the methods advocated for evaluating such interventions tend to reproduce the logics of trial assumptions, focusing on esti-mating effect sizes and controlling as far as possible for the perceived weaknesses of non-randomized designs (de Vocht et al. 2021; Craig et al. 2025). While the rise of interest in natural experiments might mitigate, to an extent, the inverse evi-dence law through generating evidence on upstream policy and environmental interventions, it reproduces the same logic: a search for average, probabilistic effects.

Trials and tribulations

On whose bodies is knowledge built? Ethics, consent, and exclusions

The dominance of trials (and quasi-experimental designs that mimic trials) has, then, overly selected for some kinds of interventions (discrete, behavioural) arriving in the evidence base and the exclusion of other kinds (upstream, structural). Yet, even for those interventions where trials are an appropriate method of choice for dem-onstrating effect, institutional methodological infrastructures serve to limit their applicability for many public health questions. These infrastructures include the organizations undertaking research (such as trial centres, universities, and global non-governmental organizations (NGOs)), their bureaucratic procedures (ethical review, research governance), and their cultures of research (such as imperatives to publish or career progressions based on generating funding). The infrastructures of medical research have a racist, colonial hinterland that has historically abused the bodies of the colonized and least powerful in society such that, as Smith (1999) put it, research is a 'dirty word' for Indigenous communities. Historical abuses, including the infamous Tuskegee experiment which left Black recruits untreated for syphilis, and the recruitment of prisoners to Phase I trials, have cast a long and dark shadow over contemporary trial recruitment. Indeed, colonial power relations continue to shape the kinds of bodies likely to be studied: contemporary large-scale trials are increasingly 'outsourced' to low-income countries where costs are lower, and recruitment is easier – often because trial participation is the only way to secure decent medical treatment, leading to what Kingori (2015) calls an 'empty choice' for participant consent.

These ongoing extractive approaches to trial recruitment continue to influence whose bodies are the source of medical knowledge and whose bodies are excluded. In the USA, where recruitment of prisoners ceased in the 1970s, the stark racial inequalities of the carceral system now mean the systematic exclusion of Black men from trial participation (Wildeman and Wang 2017). Women too are under-represented in trials. Jain et al. (2020), for instance, report on reasons for the low participation of women in Phase I trials in the USA. Those of childbearing age are excluded, with the rationale of potential risks to the foetus of drugs, compounded by poor support for those who did enrol. Such exclusions, based on normative gendered views on 'standard' physiologies, contribute to the poor evidence base for therapies for many health problems that primarily affect women and to the lack of evidence of effects of drugs on different physiologies.

There is, then, a difficult-to-manage tension between the aims of justice in terms of inclusion in trials, such that our knowledge is based on diverse and representative demographics, and the ethical imperative to ensure voluntary, informed consent. Normative exclusions, often required by ethics committees, may challenge the inclusion of those with limited capacity to understand consent processes, or children, for instance, those who may be most vulnerable to the impacts of social inequalities on health. Nkosi et al. (2022), describing the ethical challenges of including young women in an HIV intervention evaluation in South Africa, point to some of the unsettling ways in which this played out in practice, with processes such as requiring parental consent for inclusion both undermining young women's agency and threatening confidentiality. While trials and evaluations that include the voices of young women are vital in developing appropriate programmes for HIV prevention, the focus on inclusion also risks reinforcing discourses of vulnerability.

Of course, research governance in many countries has been a driver to extend representativeness in research in ethical ways, with explicit steers to include 'hard-to-reach', marginalized, or underserved populations. However, these efforts risk complex looping effects through which the demographic and social categories used by researchers (of ethnicity, or gender identity, or sexuality, for instance) may reproduce exclusionary practices. Philbin et al. (2022) take the example of young Black and Latino men who have sex with men in the USA, for whom there are often gaps in adequate HIV treatment and prevention. Here, recruitment methods and eligibility criteria are not straightforward, and the choices made by researchers do not simply have implications for sample adequacy – they also shape the very phenomena that are being described. Recruiting through gay venues and community organizations may prioritize good relations and stakeholder involvement but exclude from samples those who do not use these resources. Specifying ethnic, age, and sexuality criteria for eligibility may signal desires to include under-researched communities, but it also serves to reinforce 'at risk' or stigmatized identities. In their qualitative study, Philbin and colleagues interviewed people who would be eligible for such studies, asking about their views of recruitment. They identified inevitable mismatches between epidemiological categories and their own identities and also disquiet with eligibility criteria that singled out groups on the basis of age or other demographic factors. There are also potentials for people to misrepresent aspects of their own identities or practices to qualify for eligibility, given the small payments made for participation. As Philbin et al. note, procedural ethics and governance are, in practice, messy and contingent: consequently, so are the data that are generated through those processes.

Questions of sampling bias may be addressable in technical terms: through weighting analyses, or through careful recruitment strategies, at least for those sources of bias that are knowable. In theory, it may also be possible to design participatory trial recruitment strategies to minimize ethical risks to voluntary consent and the looping effects of creating the very categories of people that are the subject of epidemiological investigations. However, such workarounds are inevitably partial, and all too often recognized only after the event, once the research has been done. They do not address the broader limitations of reductive designs for furnishing robust evidence for what works in public health. These are rather harder to fix, and a wide range of critiques has identified key shortcomings of over-reliance on a hierarchy of evidence that places the RCT at the top. The limitations of RCTs for understanding underlying causal mechanisms have prompted a number of moves for improving the evidence base, to which critical public health scholars have contributed importantly. These include advocating for 'better trials', such as those more responsive to real-time crises such as epidemics; paying more attention to the specific contexts in which programmes are being rolled out; and calls for a greater range of evidence to be folded in to understand causal mechanisms.

Tinkering with trials

Attention to the dynamics of unfolding situations has promoted wider uptake of 'adaptive' trials, which blur the usual distinctions between trials for efficacy and for effectiveness and that include in the design the potential to adapt and learn from early findings. Montgomery (2017) traces the genealogies of adaptive designs since the 1950s and the shifting rationales mobilized by their advocates over time: from a more ethical way of doing research in early years through to a more efficient approach to research, promising to offset the risks of 'failed' trials. Although methodological development, particularly around the computational techniques needed for analysis in real time, is driven largely by pharmaceutical corporations (for personalized cancer treatments, for instance), it is in the face of global public health crises such as Ebola epidemics that public health interest has evolved.

Drawing on the development of adaptive trial design during the Ebola epidemic, in which methods were needed which not only produced robust scientific knowledge, but also provided urgent treatment in crisis, Rosengarten and Savransky (2019) note that these designs were more flexible. Some departure from the usual stringencies of methodological requirements for trials occurred, as adaptation was needed for the contingencies of unknowns in real time. They use these examples to explore the idea of 'abstraction' rather than generalization – a process of being attuned to what matters in evidence, rather than what is (universally) true. Rosengarten and Savransky (2019) suggest this is what might be needed for a 'careful biomedicine':

> The work of abstraction suggests that stabilities – the achievement of an effect in and across bodies for a period of time as may be observed in EBM – are always partial and dynamic achievements rather than mere givens. By adopting this view, there is the possibility of associating with the question of biomedical and other health interventions a form of enquiry that would neither dismiss out-right the possibility that abstractions can work in many situations, nor attempt to abstract a claim to efficacy at all costs. This is what we have tentatively called a careful biomedicine: one for which 'the best' evidence for medical practice and public health policy is evidence produced with care. [...] our proposition of a careful biomedicine suggests that the critical health field, with its persistent practices of learning to pay attention to what biomedical modes of abstraction neglect, has crucial lessons to offer to biomedicine itself. Ones that not only emphasize the latter's limitations but can also proffer alternative propositions for its transformation.
>
> (pp. 189–190)

Accounting for context: calls for methodological pluralism

Awareness that context shapes what interventions do is hardly new (Canguilhem 1991 [1949]). Yet all too often, as Shoveller et al. (2016) demonstrated in their review of how public health researchers have characterized 'context', it tends to be treated as a 'black box'. Shoveller et al. found that descriptions of context in published reports typically simply identified the setting (a country, a school) or summarized the demographics of target populations. There was little attention paid to the details that are important for understanding how interventions interact with context: relational aspects, such as the interplay between trust in institutions, stakeholders' perceptions of the intervention, and social capital. Conventional models of context posit it as simply factors external to the intervention, which should (ideally) be controlled for in evaluation. These models, suggest Shoveller and colleagues, have contributed to the poor evidence base for the transferability of interventions, which typically lacks reporting of those factors that are most likely to explain what and how interventions worked. Shoveller and colleagues acknowledge the difficulty in operationalizing what aspects of context will be relevant in any situation: knowing this requires a deep engagement with an evaluation and a more theoretical approach to thinking about how and why population health interventions work (or don't). They "suggest that it will be important to *strategically* promote research that concomitantly focuses on the roles/import of theoretically relevant contextual features and how they might substantially alter the implementation, adaptation, or potential impacts of interventions" (p. 494). This will inevitably mean drawing on a wider range of evidence – from a more interdisciplinary body of research. Shoveller et al. (2016) note:

Accepting the notion that 'Intervention = Intervention × Context' demands a new set of approaches to theory, methods, and reporting of research results of interventions within journals and elsewhere. Therefore, the fulsome pursuit of understanding context within population and public health sciences will inevitably require interdisciplinary team science approaches. This will require authentic interdisciplinary engagement, particularly with social scientists (e.g., sociologists, anthropologists), who are too often only invited to focus on the processes of implementation. A social science informed view necessarily calls into question mainstream conceptualizations of 'gold standard evidence' (i.e. the context-less RCT) and questions assumptions that data from across places and times can be combined to arrive at a transposable intervention and effect size (e.g., via meta-analyses).

(p. 496)

Calls for a greater range of disciplinary approaches and types of evidence have been a recurrent feature of critical perspectives in public health. To be sure, these are echoed in mainstream public health methodological debate. As Ogilvie et al. (2020) noted, for many public health questions, the accumulation of yet more trials all too typically results in little additional insight, given it is rare for an upstream intervention (in transport systems, or welfare, or food systems) to 'work' in any universal way. Given that effects are intricately tied to context, they suggest, better approaches are needed for evidence synthesis, which draw on a plurality of types of evidence. They draw on the metaphor of 'building a dry stone wall', which requires not standardized bricks, but careful selection and arrangements of different stones to make a robust wall. Building a useful evidence base similarly entails putting together disparate components such that the underlying functions of an intervention can be understood. Increasingly, the development of reporting guidelines for designs such as case studies used in evaluation (Shaw et al. 2023) suggests the growing openness of the public health toolbox. However, folding in various kinds of evidence – experiential knowledge, qualitative evidence – to make sense of context is to an extent perhaps a neutering of social science approaches: rather than being a source of critical perspectives, they are increasingly framed as an adjunct to the trial or the natural experiment.

Beyond linear causality

More fundamental critiques of epidemiological and RCT logic have drawn on approaches from the social sciences to think about causal logics, rather than just to 'add in' details on context and transferability. Disciplines such as development studies and philosophy have contributed to rethinking the role of trial evidence in fields such as public health. Woolcock (2013), for instance, notes that even if trials are accepted to have high internal validity, they may have limited external validity, which is the key criterion of most relevance to many decision-makers who want to know if an intervention will work in their specific patch, not whether it works in principle. Cartwright (2007, 2013) challenges many of the claims made for trials on philosophical grounds, pointing to the limitation of a design that estimates effects for a particular intervention on average for the trial population. A more important requirement for policy, she argues, is understanding the causal principles at work; that is, understanding the 'causal powers' a particular intervention mobilizes, such that we can understand whether it is likely to have similar effects elsewhere. Causal powers are capacities to change things, and key questions relate to the 'stability' (Cartwright and Munro 2010) of capacities: what can inhibit them, what fosters them, or what other capacities interact. For example, in a natural experiment evaluation of the impact of free bus travel for young people in London, UK, on the public health, Green et al. (2015) used routine data sets on young people's travel and interview data to identify the capacity of free public transport to enhance inclusivity, reduce transport poverty, and support young adults' independence, Using qualitative analysis, they identified factors essential to the stability of this capacity, including universal provision of free bus travel and a reliable bus system: this is evidence that is useful for policy actors wanting to know about whether a similar intervention is likely to have similar effects in other jurisdictions.

Critical scholars have drawn on these critiques of experimental methodologies within public health to advocate a shift away from over-reliance on the 'hypothetico-deductive' model of causality. Grant and Hood (2017), for instance, suggest this reliance has curtailed our ability to adequately research interventions in ways which provide explanations about 'what has happened'. Rod et al. (2014), echoing Cartwright's focus on causal principles, evoke what they call the 'spirit of the intervention'. They note that trials assume that interventions can be modelled as repeatable, therapeutic agents that can be separated from the social relations in which they are rolled out, rather than dynamic social processes that are difficult to capture with standardized methodologies. Drawing on their own experience of a trial of an intervention to reduce dropout and drug use amongst students, Rod and colleagues describe the challenges of forcing public health interventions into this inappropriate 'standardized' mode. They faced a 'fidelity trap': whereas the intervention was designed to be adaptable by teachers, yet measuring fidelity structured an overly routinized approach to using the intervention manual. They faced 'adaptability traps' as some staff suggested adapting the programme by introducing drug testing: an adaptation that undercut the spirit of the intervention. Implementation, they suggest, is a social process of dialogic exchange, materialized in the circulation of goods such as information between (in this case) implementers, students, and evaluators. Effectiveness is an outcome of shared, reciprocal understandings of the value of these exchanges, and evaluation requires far more nuanced accounting for how these evolve over the course of implementation Understanding how to characterize the 'spirit' of an intervention – the core principles, or mechanisms, that effect change in populations exposed to it – has been a key challenge for developments in evaluative methods and one requiring a greater range of methods, including inductive qualitative analysis (Green et al. 2015).

The 'complexity turn'

Adapting trials, taking better account of context, and incorporating qualitative evidence may well shift methodologies in more useful directions, but they do leave the normative assumptions of the conventional public health toolbox relatively untouched. The most prized evidence remains that of the probability of an effect, conceptualized as arising from a relatively linear pathway between intervention and health outcome. A more radical critique – at least in principle – has come from the so-called complexity turn (Urry 2005). Notably, many early calls for public health researchers to look to 'complexity' were rooted firmly in a discursive appeal to quantification and the natural sciences. Many accounts explicitly evoke models from physics, engineering, or ecological science. Resnicow and Page (2008), for instance, drew on metaphors from physics (quantum change, chaos, fractals) to suggest the limited purchase of rational and linear models for thinking about health behaviour and called for public health methodologies which could model complex adaptive systems, with potential tipping points. The promise of complexity metaphors for rethinking methodology has been particularly attractive in the light of seemingly intractable challenges such as health inequalities (Diez Roux 2011).

What does 'taking complexity seriously' mean for public health practice and research? Plsek and Greenhalgh (2001) first point out that health and health care are increasingly complex systems and increasingly recognized as so; that is, systems are adaptive and integrated with other systems, and there is inherent non-linearity in all systems. Despite the widespread acceptance of systems approaches, and the existence of complexity in systems, progress has been slow in terms of translating awareness of the limitations of trials into much-needed methodological development (Greenhalgh and Papoutsi 2018; Rutter et al. 2017). Taking complexity seriously also obliges us to find new metaphors for concepts such as interventions or health determinants. If systems are complex, traditional 'rainbow' models of health determinants, in which the outer ring of health determinants is illustrated as 'influencing' inner rings, down to individuals, no longer suffice: they suggest linear mechanisms and coherent pathways of causation. As Dahlgren and Whitehead have noted (2021), this illustration was never intended to suggest causal mechanisms, yet too often the rainbow model of health determinants leads us to assume layered levels, with aggregated effects imagined as flowing from the level below.

If interventions are seen as disruptions to complex systems (Hawe et al. 2009), then such mechanistic models of cause-effect are no longer helpful. 'Complex' systems are dynamic, uncertain, and non-linear. This has interrelated implications for how causal relationships are conceptualized. First, it recognizes that systems are dynamic and evolving and that any intervention, whether one introduced by a researcher in the context of a trial or one introduced in a natural experiment, such as a new tax, will in itself become part of that system. Grant and Hood (2017) highlighted the need to take actors in a system (policymakers, researchers, corporate actors) seriously in evaluations, given that they react to the intervention, shape it in response to ongoing system shifts, and seek new evidence to evaluate in real time. Findings are not, therefore, static, and it is hardly surprising that effects identified in one place and time are hard to reproduce.

A second implication is more challenging: the problem of emergence (Byrne 2013). That is, effects at one level of a system are not necessarily simply the aggregates of effects at a lower level. So, population-level effects cannot be inferred necessarily from scaling up from effects on individuals. Taking interventions to support active transport as an example, there may be 'tipping points', such as the relative safety of cycling changing as the proportion of journeys made by cycling reaches a certain point (Elvik and Bjørnskau 2017). Some effects might derive from presence or absence rather than be relative to dose: Goodman et al. (2014), for instance, documented the public health effects of free bus travel for children deriving from the fact it was universal. There may be feedback loops: for instance, congestion charging might reduce some pollution species but then increase others as private car use switches to taxis and buses (Green et al. 2020).

Methods for researching complex causation will require more than simply tweaking trial designs or adding in some qualitative context, as the very models of causality embedded in experimental methods work less well for uncovering system-wide effects or studying emergent properties of systems (Paparini et al. 2020). More recently, public health evaluations have begun to explore alternative methodological approaches from the social and political sciences, such as Qualitative Comparative Analysis (QCA) (Hanckel et al. 2021), which uses Boolean logic to investigate case series to look at contingent causality, and process tracing, which draws on close analysis of cases to make plausible inferences about causation (Johnson et al. 2025). Both have promise for generating more useful and appropriate evidence on what works, where and why to improve health and health equity, although they are underutilized to date.

Critiquing complexity

While opening up the toolbox of public health research to take into account both context and complexity holds promise for developing a more appropriate evidence base, this is hardly a panacea. Critical perspectives on the 'complexity turn' have highlighted the risks of a rather atheoretical acknowledgement of 'complexity', particularly when glossed as simply a recognition that both public health (policy) systems and the systems that shape determinants of health are both 'complicated'. Salway and Green (2017), for instance, suggest public health methodology could learn from the long histories of social science methods that have attended to structural explanations – that is, explanations of system itself, rather than the interaction of components. Further, they suggest greater folding in of public accounts, which are too often sidelined in models of systems, as they do not appear in the 'evidence' They also caution that the weak evidence base in public health for investigating complex systems is not solely an outcome of inappropriate creep of EBM methods – it is also rooted in the economic and political climates in which research is done. Salway and Green (2017) note:

Our systems analyses must be alert to: how public health problems are defined; how research questions are framed; what types of evidence are demanded; and what response options are on the table. The lack of attention to wider societal processes, and predominant focus on individual 'life-style' behaviours, as causes of health inequalities in recent years is not simply a product of medical models of evidence generation. Rather, this epistemological stance has tended to coalesce with an ideological position that locates the roots of disadvantage with individual traits and diverts attention away from policy solutions that are unpalatable to those in powerful positions.

(p. 524)

More pragmatically, others have shown that invoking 'complexity' can have political risks. Savona et al. (2021), in an analysis of industry and government documents and interviews with key stakeholders on population diets in the UK, identified the term used as what they call a 'smoke screen' to deflect any possibility of coordinated action and to devolve responsibility for poor diets to individuals.

For methodologists, there are also pragmatic risks, in that much research in public health that claims to use 'complexity' or 'system' modelling continues to rely on linear, reductive thinking. Drawing on Kwa's (2002) ideal types of 'romantic' and 'baroque' complexity (2002) in their analysis of a nutrition intervention in Australia, Warin et al. (2019) critique the 'romanticism' of models of complexity that suggest heterogeneous components (food policy, corporate interests, habits, social inequality, genetics) can be graphically integrated as if there were a coherent (if complex) 'system' that holds together. As in so many other examples, the programme they evaluated had a complex logic model of the system, yet in practice advocated individualistic health promotion to shift behaviours, with little attention to the embodied and experiential expertise of those on the receiving end. A more 'baroque' model of complexity would instead stress the local and contingent ways in which health gets done. Here, a more detailed, grounded methodology would be required: seeking not grand causal inferences, but more nuanced findings of what happens in particular places.

The contributions of Science and Technology Studies: making evidence and making publics

Methods that address the incoherence and contingencies of systems – 'baroque' accounts of systems – rather than seeking grand, unifying causal claims, are the focus of much critical scholarship in Science & Technology Studies (STS), which has increasingly turned its attention to public health over the last decades. From these perspectives, critical scholars have unpacked how the traditional toolboxes of public health do their work, and they have opened up the black box of methods to show how evidence is made in practice. Garnett (2017), for instance, attends to the work that goes into making the links between air pollution and health visible, measurable, and actionable. This is a good example of the hybridity of evidence: Garnett describes diverse sets of data, from street-side monitoring stations to meteorological modelling to hospital admissions records, and the work that goes into calibrating, integrating and stabilizing these to create meaningful patterns in data. The toxicity of air is not stable: pollutants disperse and combine, react with weather, behave unpredictably as they pass through human bodies, and do so in different ways at different points in the year. As Garnett (2017) notes, for epidemiologists, these hybrid and unstable data sources present challenges:

> ... the relationship between air pollution in the atmosphere and a human breather being exposed to this same air is neither certain nor directly measurable. This discrepancy remained problematic for the epidemiologists because they were using monitored data as proxies for human exposure.
>
> (p. 327)

Her analysis carefully depicts some of the contingencies and work that contribute to producing what appear to be coherent graphs of seasonal relationships between pollution and health effects: the data on health outcomes do not speak for themselves but require considerable skill to craft into graphs that align with seasonal variations in weather through creating appropriate time lags and models of pollution species interactions. In Garnett's example, this crafting to produce usable data required ongoing interaction between the different disciplines and data sources in the project to come to a shared, if unstable, understanding of evidence. Like much scholarship in STS, the methods here are not directed at grand claims about public health interventions, but rather at the local accomplishments of how (in this case) environmental science gets done.

From this perspective evidence gets made, rather than discovered. So, too, do the publics of public health. Taking the example of a Phase III vaginal microbicide trial in low-income settings, where medical research might be a provider of health care in a system where other provision is scarce, Montgomery and Pool (2017) show how trial infrastructures – the technologies of recruitment, consenting, counting, and recording – bring particular publics into being. Although the language of 'community engagement' suggests a pre-existing public who are the targets of public health interventions in particular places, Montgomery and Pool suggest rather that publics are 'made' by the trial, as its processes of recruitment, enrolment, and ongoing participation enact 'experimental publics', within specific local political and social contexts. Here, contexts included the stigma associated with HIV and testing; British ownership of both a major local employer and the trial funding; and gendered social and health inequalities. The trial governs the bodies of its participants through the strictures of participation: noting bodily changes; recording sexual activity; and inserting gels into vaginas. Gender exclusion from trial participation contributed to rumours about the trial, such as that it was a backdoor way for local employers to test HIV status or to undermine men's authority in the community. Montgomery and Pool (2017) suggest that:

> During its lifetime, the trial created a public of female 'biocitizens', constituted within the clinical research as informed, represented, agential. Through

procedures such as blood testing, genital examinations, and the collection of demographic and sexual behaviour data, women became governable subjects, endowed with freedom and autonomy, as specified in their signed informed consent forms.

(p. 58)

Thus, in this case, the trial creates a specific kind of public, positioning its recruits as a gendered group with capacities such as 'ability to choose' or agency. Such publics are transient and also contingent: there are no inevitable impacts of biomedical governance. Here, the context of familial and employment-based power relations intersects with the gendered inclusions and exclusions of the trial to foreground agency.

Trials also, of course, make up workers. Kingori and Gerrets (2016) explore the ways in which 'local' fieldworkers must curate particular kinds of identity in global health research projects in order to secure employment: reliable, not too educated, 'of' the community. In conditions of employment precarity and competition, locally employed fieldworkers forge identities as essential intermediaries between trial participants and principal investigators, brokers who have a vested interest in presenting local residents as hard to reach and hard to research. Drawing on examples from East African research institutes, they suggest the notion of 'pseudo data' or 'genuine fake data' to describe some of the implications of this for data generation. Fieldworkers may minimize their educational credentials or exaggerate their local connections. They may also exercise considerable agency in producing the right kind of data through changing survey questions to ones that are less likely to be offensive to local participants or changing instructions about the intervention in line with local pragmatic affordances, such as avoiding suggesting drugs should be taken with food when food is limited. Data might be constructed that were genuine in the sense that fieldworkers based the answers on their detailed knowledge of likely responses, though fake, as they were not generated through asking the prescribed questions.

Taking these insights into how methods are done in practice, Rhodes, Lancaster, and colleagues (Rhodes and Lancaster 2019; Rhodes et al. 2019) have advocated a greater attention to how public health makes its evidence, suggesting we replace a focus on evidence-based interventions with what they call 'evidence-making interventions'. This recognizes the blurred boundary between 'evidence' and 'practice', given that both are made through the local, hybrid, and contingent relations in specific places. Inevitably, implementation is messy: public health research is full of examples of interventions which work in trials but then fail when rolled out. Rather than addressing this as a problem of insufficient understanding of context or barriers to implementation, an 'evidence-making intervention' approach studies the relational and multiple nature of evidence and practice, as interventions get remade as different networks of actors perform them. The productive questions for evaluation are then around how the stability of evidence is achieved. Instead of assuming (and researching) cause-and-effect links, research might more productively document the multiple translations that happen and focus on processes, not outcomes. This is, importantly, a political as well as critical enterprise, with a focus on how things can be other, prompting speculation on how to do public health differently.

Attending to relations, not risks

Rhodes and colleagues' call for a refocus on 'evidence-making interventions' highlights the paucity of much conventional methodology for its overemphasis on single, discrete outcomes, rather than the plurality of effects that a programme or intervention can have. Without a system focus, evidence is skewed by the need for a primary outcome (reductions in smoking, fewer cases of malaria) with insufficient attention to the broader system effects of an intervention. These include not just inadvertent harms (Allen-Scott et al. 2016) and the all-too-often equity losses that accrue from well-intentioned public health interventions, but also powerful positive effects that are not detected by designs that focus on one outcome. Thus, for instance, Warbrick et al. (2016) document the widespread positive effects of a well-being intervention for Māori men that 'failed' in its narrow aim of reducing weight, and Moffatt et al. (2006) discuss the many benefits of an intervention providing welfare advice for older adults within a trial that did not identify any significant quantitative impact. Conventional trials that only demonstrate either evidence for, or no evidence for, a particular outcome tell us little about the myriad ways in which interventions can and do impact on health and on the systems that sustain or threaten it.

If a narrow focus on singular, discrete outcomes is a fundamental flaw, so too is the reification of risks, which all too often are also narrowly conceptualized and measured. Most concerning, for any research on systems, is that we are rather better at measuring the characteristics of individuals than those of societies. Rather than capturing the unequal power relations that produce ill health, our data sources provide measures of individual-level risk factors: income, race, or gender. These too often become reified as if they were the cause of some outcome, located in the person, not an indicator of unequal relationships of class, racism, and other structures.

Intersectionality

Attending to intersectionality is one way in which critical public health scholars have approached the limitations of individual-level measures. As Persmark et al. (2020) explain, in their analysis of intersections that might trouble a story of prescription opioid misuse (POM), indicators of ethnicity, income, gender, and so on can be conceptualized as:

> proxies for social positions within complex, interlocking systems of inequality and the social experiences that these positions likely entail. Observed inequalities in POM across strata are therefore understood to be an end result of intersectional social processes operating at several ecological levels.
>
> (p. 399)

Persmark et al. found that, although the opioid crisis was largely characterized as one affecting White populations, there were intersections of the population (for instance, high-income African American women) who were also affected, yet invisible in narratives of the crisis.

In a similar vein, Ferlatte et al. (2018) note that in Canada, gay, bisexual, and other men who have sex with men (GBM) have experienced the brunt of the HIV epidemic and that solutions remain largely focused on behaviour, not the intersecting dynamics of structures that shape the risks they face. Taking first the concept of syndemics (Singer and Clair 2003) – the notion that multiple epidemics affect marginalized communities in ways that are synergistic – they note that GBM are at the crux of multiple epidemics related to social exclusion and stigma. The individual-level factors that are typically associated with HIV exposure in standard epidemiological studies (polydrug use, intimate partner violence, mental health problems, for instance) are highly correlated with each other. Rather than representing behavioural risks, these can be conceptualized as indicators of social marginalization, that is, as representing the health outcomes of unequal relations of power. As Ferlatte et al. note, though, men who have sex with men are not a homogenous group: there are also cross-cutting relations of social inequality by ethnicity, geography, social class, and age. Here, they turn to intersectional theory to identify sub-groups of the GBM population that might be particularly at risk of syndemics. They outline the aims of drawing together intersectional theory into quantitative analysis:

> Quantitative intersectional analyses contrast with unitary mainstream public health research and those typically used in syndemic research by highlighting diversity as well as patterns. In unitary studies demographic variables are seen as having an 'additive effect' … and the independent effects of each social category are computed and layered (e.g., the independent effect of being a man in addition to the independent effect of being gay, etc.). By contrast, quantitative intersectional studies aim to uncover interactions of social categories on health or social outcomes.
>
> (p. 511)

Using an intersectional approach, they identified sub-groups that were at particular risk of syndemics of psycho-social issues that are associated with sex without a condom, including those who were single or partnered with men, rather than those partnered with women, those of Indigenous ancestry, and those with lower incomes. Identifying sub-groups using intersectional approaches to the analysis also identified important variations: for younger men (under 30), there was no protective effect of a female partner.

However, such attempts at ever-finer segregations of the categories we use in public health research also risk reifying and solidifying 'identities' as if these sub-categories shared particular sets of risks or positions. This matters for the interventions we develop. Mulinari et al. (2018) contrast the use of such 'categorical' approaches with 'anti-categorical' approaches to intersectionality in their analysis of ethnic and racial differences in the take-up of seasonal influenza vaccination in the USA. While 'anti-categorical' approaches tend to be used more in qualitative social science, founded on critiques of categorization in a messy and hybrid world, Mulinari et al. (2018) also highlight limitations using quantitative analysis. Using an analysis of discriminatory accuracy, they show that variation between sub-groups is significant and that ethnic/racial aggregation has overemphasized the differences between groups. As they note, this matters for public health interventions, given that targeting and tailoring may be unjustified on scientific grounds, as well as risking further stigmatizing some sub-groups and further eroding trust in public health institutions. Categories constructed from ever-smaller taxonomies may reflect social structural intersections, but they are unlikely to be useful for informing individual-level interventions. Mulinari et al. also note the continued emphasis by the Centers for Disease Control and Prevention (CDC) on reporting outcomes such as vaccination by ethnicity and the more limited focus on other axes of inequality: political decisions about which categories are researched, and with what consequences, become solidified and part of the taken-for-granted infrastructure of doing public health research. This was also a core finding of Shim's (2014) work on heart disease in the USA. The histories of epidemiological study have reified 'race' as a variable to measure, categorized as White/Black, as if this was a property of individuals, not a relation in a specific world, and one that intersects with class and gender.

Epistemic justice

Underpinning the tensions of attending to power differentials without simultaneously reinforcing them is a broader problem facing public health methodologies: that of epistemic (in)justice. That is, our methods routinely sideline, ignore, or discount the kinds of knowledge produced by those marginalized by structures of power. Indigenous and southern knowledge is reduced to 'beliefs' (Bhakuni and Abimbola 2021), experiential knowledge is included only at the margins, and knowledge from the global south is systematically downplayed through the institutions of global health and knowledge production outlined in Chapter 1. Within northern public health, epistemic inequalities arise from the limited pool of recruits to health research and the paucity of participatory approaches. There have been calls for explicit anti-racist approaches (Rai et al. 2024) that widen this pool, build trust and reciprocity with communities, and challenge white privilege. Drawing on, and in conversation with, the writings of bell hooks and others, Petteway's (2023a) poem *RELATIVES//Risks or, I am not your data: Ode to Delphrine's walk, pt. II* references hooks' concept of 'homeplace', where "all black people could strive to be subjects, not objects, where we could be affirmed in our minds and hearts … where we could restore to ourselves the dignity denied us on the outside in the public world" (hooks 2015, p. 42). Petteway (2023a, p. 2, reprinted by permission of Informa UK Limited, trading as Taylor & Francis Group, www.tandfonline.com) writes:

> I am a great nephew
> I am a proud son
> I am a blossom,
> the new fruit
> from a seed
> dropped long ago,
> and rooted –
>   I am not your data.

Petteway (2023b) unpacks the ways in which public health methodologies have been implicated in the othering of Black communities in the USA and the erasure of their knowledge: matters of "epistemic, procedural, and distributive justice that undergird epidemiological knowledge production related to racial health inequities in the U.S." (2023b, p. 5). He draws on Black feminist philosopher Kristie Dotson's (2011) conceptualization of 'epistemic violence' to critique 'extractivist' methods of epidemiology, its reductionism, and the colour-blind gaze of White researchers.

Questions of epistemic injustice are neither solved by taking a complexity approach, nor by simply adding in qualitative methods to the toolbox of public health research (Bowleg 2017). It is not that experiential knowledge, or public accounts, or Indigenous knowledge do not exist: there is a wealth of evidence from participatory research, anthropology, sociology, and other many sources that documents public understandings, priorities, and desires. There is also a growing recognition that such evidence should be synthesized and available for public health policy. Yet the greater incorporation of these sources in systematic reviews and guidelines has not, to date, significantly shifted public health policymaking. Colvin (2022), reflecting on technical work with a WHO guidelines group, notes that moves towards system thinking, and incorporating ethnographic evidence syntheses, made only incremental changes to the ways in which interventions were conceptualized. When such evidence is simply folded in within dominant (reductionist, linear) paradigms, it fails to shift initial framings of the problem and its potential solutions. As Bodini et al. (2020) suggest, in their review of methodological challenges of researching with activists, incorporating marginalized sources of knowing requires "exposing research design, methods, and analysis to a range of different perspectives" (p. 388) that actors normally excluded can bring. This requires new ways of doing research, beyond tinkering with trials, and ones which go beyond simply measuring what Cornish (2021) terms the 'poor and arrogant concepts' of success or failure.

Conclusion

The place for critical scholars in advocating for novel methods or approaches is, perhaps, an inevitably awkward one. Hierarchies of credibility will always favour evidence and explanations that go with the grain of established wisdom and utilize conventional methodologies. Doing research that challenges established thinking demands at times a higher standard of proof. If the findings of a study go against the grain, using less conventional methodologies provides an easy target for critics, rejecting the message on grounds of validity. However, this risks a conservatism of methodology: as Green and Speed (2018) put it, the tempting choice is to:

> … batten down the hatches, retreating to the established practices of traditional scholarly approaches: more extensive peer review; demanding higher standards of evidence for arguments; perhaps become more cautious of publishing papers that are likely to be subjected to similar critique. In essence, to engage in the

mary rituals that delineate the boundaries between 'science' and 'non-science' so that the findings are seen to be firmly 'scientific'.

(pp. 129–130)

Yet, this reliance on the conventions of method to shore up unpalatable findings has its own risks: reifying the rituals of validation even further, and, for instance, consolidating hierarchical assumptions about journals which position those of the anglophone global north as prestigious, and others as marginal, 'predatory', and of low value. In a *Critical Public Health* editorial of 2014, Green noted that despite considerable critique of the limitations of over-reliance on trial evidence and the complexity turn, there had perhaps been less progress than needed on developing methods for making useful and robust public health evidence (Green 2014). Asking 'what kind of research does public health need?' the editorial suggested four key domains: research that examined affect as well as effect; research that takes systems (and the interlocking networks that make them up) seriously; emphasis on process as much as outcomes; and development of an ethos of public health research that is more reflexive about its politics and ethics. In the decade since, there has been some progress on much of this agenda: public health does take systems seriously, and there have been methodological developments that have widened the evidence base for what works in public health. Yet, the struggle for epistemic justice remains.

References

Allen-Scott, L.K. *et al.* (2016) 'Operationalizing the "population health" approach to permit consideration and minimization of unintended harms of public health interventions: a malaria control example', *Critical Public Health*, 26(3), pp. 244–257. Available at: https://doi.org/10.1080/09581596.2014.980397

Bell, K (2012) 'Cochrane reviews and the behavioural turn in evidence-based medicine', *Health Sociology Review*, 21(3), pp. 313–321. Available at: https://doi.org/10.5172/hesr.2012.21.3.313

Bhakuni, H. and Abimbola, S. (2021) 'Epistemic injustice in academic global health', *The Lancet Global Health*, 9(10), pp. e1465–e1470. Available at: https://doi.org/10.1016/S2214-109X(21)00301-6

Bodini, C. *et al.* (2020) 'Methodological challenges in researching activism in action: civil society engagement towards health for all', *Critical Public Health*, 30(4), pp. 386–397. Available at: https://doi.org/10.1080/09581596.2019.1650892

Borozdna, E. (2023) 'Evidence-based medicine and physicians' institutional agency in Russian clinical settings', *Critical Public Health*, 33(4), pp. 409–420. Available at: https://doi.org/10.1080/09581596.2023.2180608

Bowleg, L. (2017) 'Towards a critical health equity research stance: why epistemology and methodology matter more than qualitative methods', *Health Education & Behavior*, 44(5), pp. 677–684. Available at: https://doi.org/10.1177/1090198117728760

Byrne, D. (2013) 'Evaluating complex social interventions in a complex world', *Evaluation*, 19(3), pp. 217–228. Available at: https://doi.org/10.1177/1356389013495617

Canguilhem, G. (1991) [1949] *The normal and the pathological*. New York: Zone Books.

Cartwright, N. (2007) 'Are RCTs the gold standard?', *BioSocieties*, 2(1), pp. 11–20. Available at: https://doi.org/10.1017/S1745855207005029

Cartwright, N. (2013) 'Knowing what we are talking about: why evidence doesn't always travel', *Evidence and Policy*, 9(1), pp. 97–112. Available at: https://doi.org/10.1332/174426413X662581

Cartwright, N. and Munro, E. (2010) 'The limitations of randomized controlled trials in predicting effectiveness', *Journal of Evaluation in Clinical Practice*, 16(2), pp. 260–266. Available at: https://doi.org/10.1111/j.1365-2753.2010.01382.x

Colvin, C.J. (2022) 'Understanding global health policy engagements with qualitative research: qualitative evidence syntheses and the OptimizeMNH guidelines', *Social Science & Medicine*, 300, p. 114678. Available at: https://doi.org/10.1016/j.socscimed.2021.114678

Cornish, F. (2021) '"Grenfell changes everything?" Activism beyond hope and despair', *Critical Public Health*, 31(3), pp. 293–305. Available at: https://doi.org/10.1080/09581596.2020.1869184

Craig, P. *et al.* (2022) 'Making better use of natural experimental evaluation in population health', *BMJ*, p. e070872. Available at: https://doi.org/10.1136/bmj-2022-070872

Craig, P. *et al.* (2025). 'Using natural experiments to evaluate population health and health system interventions: new framework for producers and users of evidence', *BMJ*, 388. https://doi.org/10.1136/bmj-2024-080505

Dahlgren, G. and Whitehead, M. (2021) 'The Dahlgren-Whitehead model of health determinants: 30 years on and still chasing rainbows', *Public Health*, 199, pp. 20–24. Available at: https://doi.org/10.1016/j.puhe.2021.08.009

De Vocht, F. *et al.* (2021) 'Conceptualising natural and quasi experiments in public health', *BMC Medical Research Methodology*, 21(1), p. 32. Available at: https://doi.org/10.1186/s12874-021-01224-x

Diez Roux, A.V. (2011) 'Complex systems thinking and current impasses in health disparities research', *American Journal of Public Health*, 101(9), pp. 1627–1634. Available at: https://doi.org/10.2105/AJPH.2011.300149

Dotson, K. (2011) 'Tracking epistemic violence, tracking practices of silencing', *Hypatia*, 26(2), pp. 236–257. Available at: https://doi.org/10.1111/j.1527-2001.2011.01177.x

Elvik, R. and Bjørnskau, T. (2017) 'Safety-in-numbers: a systematic review and meta-analysis of evidence', *Safety Science*, 92, pp. 274–282. Available at: https://doi.org/10.1016/j.ssci.2015.07.017

Ferlatte, O. *et al.* (2018) 'Combining intersectionality and syndemic theory to advance understandings of health inequities among Canadian gay, bisexual and other men who have sex with men', *Critical Public Health*, 28(5), pp. 509–521. Available at: https://doi.org/10.1080/09581596.2017.1380298

Garnett, E. (2017) 'Enacting toxicity: epidemiology and the study of air pollution for public health', *Critical Public Health*, 27(3), pp. 325–336. Available at: https://doi.org/10.1080/09581596.2017.1302562

Goodman, A. *et al.* (2014) '"We can all just get on a bus and go": rethinking independent mobility in the context of the universal provision of free bus travel to young Londoners', *Mobilities*, 9(2), pp. 275–293. Available at: https://doi.org/10.1080/17450101.2013.782848

Grant, R.L. and Hood, R. (2017) 'Complex systems, explanation and policy: implications of the crisis of replication for public health research', *Critical Public Health*, 27(5), pp. 525–532. Available at: https://doi.org/10.1080/09581596.2017.1282603

Green, C.P., Heywood, J.S. and Navarro Paniagua, M. (2020) 'Did the London congestion charge reduce pollution?', *Regional Science and Urban Economics*, 84, p. 103573. Available at: https://doi.org/10.1016/j.regsciurbeco.2020.103573

Green, J. (2014) 'What kind of research does public health need?', *Critical Public Health*, 24(3). pp. 249–252. Available at: https://doi.org/10.1080/09581596.2014.917813

Green, J. and Speed, E. (2018) 'Critical analysis, credibility, and the politics of publishing in an era of "fake news" ', *Critical Public Health*, 28(2), pp. 129–131. Available at: https://doi.org/10.1080/09581596.2017.1421597

Green, J. *et al.* (2015) 'Integrating quasi-experimental and inductive designs in evaluation: a case study of the impact of free bus travel on public health', *Evaluation*, 21(4), pp. 391–406. Available at: https://doi.org/10.1177/1356389015605205

Green, J. *et al.* (2022) 'The publics of public health: learning from COVID-19', *Critical Public Health*, 32(5), pp. 592–599. Available at: https://doi.org/10.1080/09581596.2022.2077701

Greenhalgh, T. (2020) 'Will COVID-19 be evidence-based medicine's nemesis?', *PLOS Medicine*, 17(6), p. e1003266. Available at: https://doi.org/10.1371/journal.pmed.1003266

Greenhalgh, T. and Papoutsi, C. (2018) 'Studying complexity in health services research: desperately seeking an overdue paradigm shift', *BMC Medicine*, 16(1), pp. 95, s12916-018-1089-4. Available at: https://doi.org/10.1186/s12916-018-1089-4

Hanckel, B. *et al.* (2021) 'The use of Qualitative Comparative Analysis (QCA) to address causality in complex systems: a systematic review of research on public health interventions', *BMC Public Health*, 21(1), p. 877. Available at: https://doi.org/10.1186/s12889-021-10926-2

Hawe, P., Shiell, A. and Riley, T. (2009) 'Theorising interventions as events in systems', *American Journal of Community Psychology*, 43(3–4), pp. 267–276. Available at: https://doi.org/10.1007/s10464-009-9229-9

Herrick, C. and Bell, K. (2024) 'The social life of natural experiments in epidemiology and public health', *Sociology of Health & Illness*, 46(2), pp. 276–294. Available at: https://doi.org/10.1111/1467-9566.13703.

hooks, b (2015) *Yearning: race, gender, and cultural politics.* New York London: Routledge. Available at: https://doi.org/10.4324/9781315743110

Jain, N., Cottingham, M.D. and Fisher, J.A. (2020) 'Disadvantaged, outnumbered, and discouraged: women's experiences as healthy volunteers in U.S. Phase I trials', *Critical Public Health*, 30(2), pp. 141–152. Available at: https://doi.org/10.1080/09581596.2018.1529861

Johnson, R., Beach, D. and Al-Janabi, H. (2025) 'How is process tracing applied in health research? A systematic scoping review', *Social Science & Medicine*, 366, p. 117539. Available at: https://doi.org/10.1016/j.socscimed.2024.117539

Kingori, P. (2015) 'The "empty choice": a sociological examination of choosing medical research participation in resource-limited sub-Saharan Africa', *Current Sociology*, 63(5), pp. 763–778. Available at: https://doi.org/10.1177/0011392115590093

Kingori, P. and Gerrets, R. (2016) 'Morals, morale and motivations in data fabrication: medical research fieldworkers views and practices in two sub-Saharan African contexts', *Social Science & Medicine*, 166, pp. 150–159. Available at: https://doi.org/10.1016/j.socscimed.2016.08.019

Knaapen, L. (2013) 'Being "evidence-based" in the absence of evidence: the management of non-evidence in guideline development', *Social Studies of Science*, 43(5), pp. 681–706. Available at: https://doi.org/10.1177/0306312713483679

Kwa, C. (2002) 'Romantic and baroque conceptions of complex wholes in the sciences', in Law, J., *Complexities*. Edited by A. Mol. Duke University Press, pp. 23–52. Available at: https://doi.org/10.1215/9780822383550-002

Moffatt, S. *et al.* (2006) 'Using quantitative and qualitative data in health services research – what happens when mixed method findings conflict? [ISRCTN61522618]', *BMC Health Services Research*, 6(1), p. 28. Available at: https://doi.org/10.1186/1472-6963-6-28

Montgomery, C.M. (2017) 'From standardization to adaptation: clinical trials and the moral economy of anticipation', *Science as Culture*, 26(2), pp. 232–254. Available at: https://doi.org/10.1080/09505431.2016.1255721

Montgomery, C.M. and Pool, R. (2017) 'From "trial community" to "experimental publics": how clinical research shapes public participation', *Critical Public Health*, 27(1), pp. 50–62. Available at: https://doi.org/10.1080/09581596.2016.1212161

Mulinari, S. *et al.* (2018) 'Categorical and anti-categorical approaches to US racial/ethnic groupings: revisiting the National 2009 H1N1 Flu Survey (NHFS)', *Critical Public Health*, 28(2), pp. 177–189. Available at: https://doi.org/10.1080/09581596.2017.1316831

Mykhalovskiy, E. and Weir, L. (2004) 'The problem of evidence-based medicine: directions for social science', *Social Science & Medicine*, 59(5), pp. 1059–1069. Available at: https://doi.org/10.1016/j.socscimed.2003.12.002

Nkosi, B. *et al.* (2022) 'Putting research ethics in context: rethinking vulnerability and agency within a research ethics case study on HIV prevention for young girls in South Africa', *SSM – Qualitative Research in Health*, 2, p. 100081. Available at: https://doi.org/10.1016/j.ssmqr.2022.100081

Ogilvie, D. (2005) 'Systematic reviews of health effects of social interventions: 2. Best available evidence: how low should you go?', *Journal of Epidemiology & Community Health*, 59(10), pp. 886–892. Available at: https://doi.org/10.1136/jech.2005.034199

Ogilvie, D. *et al.* (2020) 'Making sense of the evidence in population health intervention research: building a dry stone wall', *BMJ Global Health*, 5(12), p. e004017. Available at: https://gh.bmj.com/content/5/12/e004017

Owusu-Addo, E., Cross, R. and Sarfo-Mensah, P. (2017) 'Evidence-based practice in local public health service in Ghana', *Critical Public Health*, 27(1), pp. 125–138. Available at: https://doi.org/10.1080/09581596.2016.1182621

Paparini, S. *et al.* (2020) 'Case study research for better evaluations of complex interventions: rationale and challenges', *BMC Medicine*, 18(1), p. 301. Available at: https://doi.org/10.1186/s12916-020-01777-6

Pearce, W. and Raman, S. (2014) 'The new randomised controlled trials (RCT) movement in public policy: challenges of epistemic governance', *Policy Sciences*, 47(4), pp. 387–402. Available at: https://doi.org/10.1007/s11077-014-9208-3

Persmark, A. *et al.* (2020) 'Intersectional inequalities and the U.S. opioid crisis: challenging dominant narratives and revealing heterogeneities', *Critical Public Health*, 30(4), pp. 398–414. Available at: https://doi.org/10.1080/09581596.2019.1626002

Petteway, R. (2023a) 'RELATIVES//Risks or, I am not your data: Ode to Delphrine's walk, pt. II', *Critical Public Health*, 33(1), pp. 1–4. Available at: https://doi.org/10.1080/09581596.2022.2096429

Petteway, R. (2023b) 'On epidemiology as racial-capitalist (re)colonization and epistemic violence', *Critical Public Health*, 33(1), pp. 5–12. Available at: https://doi.org/10.1080/09581596.2022.2107486

Philbin, M.M. *et al.* (2022) 'How Black and Latino young men who have sex with men in the United States experience and engage with eligibility criteria and recruitment practices: implications for the sustainability of community-based research', *Critical Public Health*, 32(5), pp. 677–688. Available at: https://doi.org/10.1080/09581596.2021.1918329

Phillips, G. and Green, J. (2015) 'Working for the public health: politics, localism and epistemologies of practice', *Sociology of Health & Illness*, 37(4), pp. 491–505. Available at: https://doi.org/10.1111 /1467-9566.12214

Plsek, P.E. and Greenhalgh, T. (2001) 'Complexity science: the challenge of complexity in health care', *BMJ*, 323(7313), pp. 625–628. Available at: https://doi.org/10.1136/bmj.323.7313.625

Pope, C. (2003) 'Resisting evidence: the study of evidence-based medicine as a contemporary social movement', *Health: An Interdisciplinary Journal for the Social Study of Health, Illness and Medicine*, 7(3), pp. 267–282. Available at: https://doi.org/10.1177/1363459303007003002

Rai, T. *et al.* (2024) 'How should we do racially just research? Learning from a qualitative study on COVID-19 pandemic experiences in the UK', *Journal of Critical Public Health*, 1(2), pp. 24–42. Available at: https://doi.org/10.55016/ojs/jcph.v1i2.77774

Resnicow, K. and Page, S.E. (2008) 'Embracing chaos and complexity: a quantum change for public health', *American Journal of Public Health*, 98(8), pp. 1382–1389. Available at: https://doi.org/10.2105 /AJPH.2007.129460

Rhodes, T. and Lancaster, K. (2019) 'Evidence-making interventions in health: a conceptual framing', *Social Science & Medicine*, 238, p. 112488. Available at: https://doi.org/10.1016/j.socscimed.2019.112488

Rhodes, T., Lancaster, K. and Rosengarten, M. (2020) 'A model society: maths, models and expertise in viral outbreaks', *Critical Public Health*, 30(3), pp. 253–256. Available at: https://doi.org/10.1080 /09581596.2020.1748310

Rhodes, T. *et al.* (2019) 'Evidence-making controversies: the case of hepatitis C treatment and the promise of viral elimination', *Critical Public Health*, 29(3), pp. 260–273. Available at: https://doi.org/10.1080 /09581596.2018.1459475

Rod, M.H. *et al.* (2014) 'The spirit of the intervention: reflections on social effectiveness in public health intervention research', *Critical Public Health*, 24(3), pp. 296–307. Available at: https://doi.org/10.1080 /09581596.2013.841313

Rosengarten, M. and Savransky, M. (2019) 'A careful biomedicine? Generalization and abstraction in RCTs', *Critical Public Health*, 29(2), pp. 181–191. Available at: https://doi.org/10.1080/09581596.2018.1431387

Rutter, H. *et al.* (2017) 'The need for a complex systems model of evidence for public health', *The Lancet*, 390(10112), pp. 2602–2604. Available at: https://doi.org/10.1016/S0140-6736(17)31267-9

Salway, S. and Green, J. (2017) 'Towards a critical complex systems approach to public health', *Critical Public Health*, 27(5), pp. 523–524. Available at: https://doi.org/10.1080/09581596.2017.1368249

Savona, N. *et al.* (2021) '"Complexity" as a rhetorical smokescreen for UK public health inaction on diet', *Critical Public Health*, 31(5), pp. 510–520. Available at: https://doi.org/10.1080/09581596.2020.1755421

Shaw, S.E. *et al.* (2023) 'TRIPLE C reporting principles for case study evaluations of the role of context in complex interventions', *BMC Medical Research Methodology*, 23(1), p. 115. Available at: https://doi.org /10.1186/s12874-023-01888-7

Shim, J.K. (2014) *Heart-sick: the politics of risk, inequality, and heart disease*. New York: New York University Press.

Shoveller, J. *et al.* (2016) 'A critical examination of representations of context within research on population health interventions', *Critical Public Health*, 26(5), pp. 487–500. Available at: https://doi.org/10.1080 /09581596.2015.1117577

Singer, M. and Clair, S. (2003) 'Syndemics and public health: reconceptualizing disease in bio-social context', *Medical Anthropology Quarterly*, 17(4), pp. 423–441. Available at: https://doi.org/10.1525 /maq.2003.17.4.423

Smith, G.D. and Ebrahim, S. (2001) 'Epidemiology—is it time to call it a day?', *International Journal of Epidemiology*, 30(1), pp. 1–11. Available at: https://doi.org/10.1093/ije/30.1.1

Smith, L. T. (1999). *Decolonizing methodologies: Research and indigenous peoples.* London: Zed Books.

Stevens, A. (2011) 'Telling policy stories: An ethnographic study of the use of evidence in policy-making in the UK', *Journal of Social Policy*, 40(2), pp. 237–255. Available at: https://doi.org/10.1017 /S0047279410000723

Urry, J. (2005) 'The Complexity Turn', *Theory, Culture & Society*, 22(5), pp. 1–14. Available at: https://doi.org/10.1177/0263276405057188

Warbrick, I. *et al.* (2016) 'The biopolitics of Māori biomass: towards a new epistemology for Māori health in Aotearoa/New Zealand', *Critical Public Health*, 26(4), pp. 394–404. Available at: https://doi.org/10.1080 /09581596.2015.1096013

Warin, M. and Zivkovic, T. (2019) *Fatness, Obesity, and Disadvantage in the Australian Suburbs: Unpalatable Politics.* Cham: Springer International Publishing. Available at: https://doi.org/10.1007 /978-3-030-01009-6

Wieringa, S. *et al.* (2021) 'Clinical guidelines and the pursuit of reducing epistemic uncertainty. An ethnographic study of guideline development panels in three countries', *Social Science & Medicine*, 272, p. 113702. Available at: https://doi.org/10.1016/j.socsci med.2021.113702

Wildeman, C. and Wang, E.A. (2017) 'Mass incarceration, public health, and widening inequality in the USA', *The Lancet*, 389(10077), pp. 1464–1474. Available at: https://doi. org/10.1016 /S0140-6736(17)30259-3

Woolcock, M. (2013) 'Using case studies to explore the external validity of "complex" development interventions', *Evaluation*, 19(3), pp. 229–248. Available at: https://doi.org/ 10.1177/1356389013495210

3 Public health, medicalization, and biomedicalization

There is, and has long been, an uneasy relationship between public health and clinical medicine (hereafter, medicine).[1] This stems from their overlapping institutional histories yet distinct orientations and goals, with medicine having a downstream, individualized focus and public health focusing, at least ostensibly, on the upstream conditions that cause populations to be sick in the first place (e.g. see McLaren et al. 2024a). This relationship and its corresponding tensions have long preoccupied critical public health scholars concerned with the professional, sectoral, and epistemic power of medicine, including the ways in which medicine's dominance obscures and distracts from meaningful attention to systemic causes of poor health and their highly inequitable distribution (Green and Labonté 2008; Valles 2018).

This chapter considers important recent scholarship on how processes of medicalization and biomedicalization have shaped the field of public health. It first grounds the chapter in the long-standing framework of *medicalization*, which continues to be highly pertinent to debates in public health research, scholarship, practice, and policy. It then discusses a relatively more recent focus on processes of *biomedicalization* and the conceptual lens that emerged from scholars' (primarily medical sociologists') observations that medicalization was theoretically insufficient to account for dramatic recent techno-scientific changes in health and medicine and the complex ways in which medicine and society are co-constituted. The chapter concludes with some thoughts around de-medicalizing, and re-politicizing, the field of public health.

Medicalization

With attribution to medical sociologist Zola's work in the early 1970s, Clarke et al. (2003) describe *medicalization* as a set of processes whereby aspects of life previously outside of the jurisdiction of medicine come to be defined and treated as medical problems. Described as a 'regime of truth' due to the cultural authority and hegemony of medicine, medicalization has been a significant framework for understanding and illuminating the nature of relations between medicine and society for over fifty years (Neresini et al. 2019).

DOI: 10.4324/9781003654650-4

Focusing on the US context, Clarke et al. (2003) describe medicalization as the second key social transformation in how healing and curing were institutionally positioned in society. The first transformation, which Clarke et al. (2003) argue made medicalization possible, was the clinical, scientific, technological, and institutional rise and establishment of a profession of medicine between around 1890 and 1945. Then, due to major investments in medical knowledge and clinical interventions during the post-Second World War period, the medical profession gained significant political, economic, and sociocultural status, thus setting the stage for its jurisdictional and cultural expanse into other domains of life. Early examples involved the medicalization of so-called moral problems such as drug or alcohol use. Later, the rise of pharmaceutical and medical technology industries under early neoliberal capitalism led to medicalization of, for example, childbirth and menopause in the 1970s and of post-traumatic stress disorder and attention deficit hyperactivity disorder in the 1980s and 1990s. Well-established and well-theorized consequences of medicalization include pathologizing normal behaviour, disempowering individuals in care contexts, decontextualizing peoples' experiences, and depoliticizing social concerns (Clarke et al. 2003; Crawford 1980).

Medicalization and public health

Processes of medicalization have long preoccupied critical scholars in public health. Indeed, in a recent piece, Schrecker (2022) identifies "the potentially pernicious impact of medicalization and the dominance of medical frames of reference" (p. 139) as one of five key elements of a critical public health perspective. Echoing important arguments made much earlier by Crawford (1980), Schrecker (2022) describes medicalization as entailing a narrow focus on individual situations that are better understood as consequences of macro-scale political and economic forces and choices. Bringing a global public health lens, Clark (2014) provides a succinct description of medicalization as a process characterized by *reductionism* – ignoring or excluding context and reducing explanations to physical or biological realms; *individualism* – placing responsibility and often blame on individuals rather than with structures that shape behaviours and experiences; and *technological bias* – favouring drugs, devices, or other technologies, usually for curative purposes. These elements reflect and are perpetuated by neoliberal political economic ideology, which is likewise premised on individualized, technical solutions to problems (see also Chapter 1 and Chapter 6 in this volume).

As described by Clark (2014), manifestations of medicalization in public health include an overemphasis on the role of health care to health and a tendency to elevate the role and status of medical professionals in health. Both manifestations are inconsistent with what is known about upstream determinants of health (see also Chapter 4 in this volume), and they serve to obstruct socio-structural approaches to understanding and redressing health inequities. Medicalization processes also manifest in the elevation of hierarchies of scientific evidence that treat certain kinds of evidence – such as evidence from randomized controlled trials (RCTs) as gold standards, when in fact they are highly inappropriate to scenarios where causal processes are complex, dynamic, and multiple (see Chapter 2 in this volume). Illustrative of the reach of these epistemic dynamics of medicalization is political economy of health scholars Chernomas' and Hudson's (2019) critical analysis of the Nobel Prize-winning work of economist Esther Duflo, which conceptualizes major problems in development economics – like global poverty – as rooted in poor choices by individuals. Duflo's RCT-based research aims to incentivize better decisions by individuals, such as spending their limited money on better food choices. It thereby obscures structural causes of poverty, which lie in political and economic decisions made by people and institutions who wield immense power.

Medicalization of public health – recent scholarly examples

Examples of medicalization processes shaping public health are numerous; the COVID-19 pandemic provides a recent example. In their editorial to accompany a Special Section of *Critical Public Health* focused on COVID-19, Marelli et al. (2022) remark on the 'array of technological solutions' that arose to reduce the spread of COVID-19, such as digital contact tracing and exposure-notification technologies. This occurred despite the underwhelming effectiveness of these solutions (especially relative to their 'silver bullet' allure) and their problematic tendencies to omit contextual factors, obscure alternative solutions, and exacerbate social inequities. Marelli et al. (2022) further point out that this 'COVID-19 techno-solutionism' often relied on an obscure mix of public–private partnerships, thus illustrating the close alliance noted above between medicalization and neoliberal political economy. That alliance raises important questions around the transparency (or lack thereof) of decision-making processes and the implications of relying on private companies (such as Google) for software application development that is heavily subsidized by public money, namely the question of who benefits from such arrangements. Others, writing in popular forums (Hancock et al. 2020; McLaren and Hennessy 2020), have likewise noted that while the COVID-19 pandemic brought public health into the spotlight, it advanced a narrow, medicalized version of public health where certain types of experts (physicians) and ways of knowing (epidemiology, virology) were prominent, thus serving to obscure the dynamics of power and politics that fundamentally shaped the pandemic, including its highly inequitable impacts.

Indeed, one important illustration of the extent and ways in which processes of medicalization have shaped the field of public health is that the phrase 'public health' itself has, in some contexts, come to signify the reductionist, individualized, and technological orientation emblematic of medicalization. This can be seen in critical analyses of issues framed as 'public health problems'. Alexander et al. (2014), for example, analysed the emergence of children's active play as a *public health issue* in Canada. This emergence, according to the authors, occurred in the context of growing concern about a so-called childhood obesity epidemic that is believed to be caused by declining physical activity.

Based on a discourse analysis of documents from Canadian public health websites, and guided by Bacchi's question-posing approach, Alexander et al.

(2014) identified several assumptions and practices embedded in the public health discourse on active play, which are illustrative of processes of medicalization. The first is that play is viewed in public health materials as a productive activity that is undertaken for the purpose of energy expenditure, with the intent to curb rising levels of obesity. This productivity frame – consistent with the neoliberal allegiance of medicalization processes – serves also to highlight economic benefits of play, with respect to rising health care costs. A second characteristic of public health discourse on active play identified by the authors was that tropes of 'fun' and 'pleasure' were mobilized to promote physical activity, thus conveying a reductive and potentially exclusionary assumption that being active and having fun necessarily co-exist for all children (Alexander et al. 2014).

The third is that the public health framing of active play encouraged children to self-govern their own leisure time to promote their health. Examples of self-governance mechanisms included workbooks for children to monitor and evaluate their own active play, as well as encouragements for children to have 'active friends'. Alexander et al. (2014) conclude that the public health framing places 'discursive limits' on the issue of active play. These discursive limits serve to privilege some versions of the issue – i.e. a narrative of active play as a risk factor in an epidemic of obesity, for which individuals and families are responsible – over others that may in fact resonate far more closely with the lives of publics.

As a second illustration, Riemann (2019) considers the medicalization processes that can occur when violence is framed as a public health problem. They do so through a critical analysis of a US-based violence prevention initiative called *Cure Violence*. That initiative was launched by a former World Health Organization (WHO) epidemiologist who argued that violence is an actual (not metaphorical) disease, which can be controlled and contained via epidemiologic methods and intervention by health care professionals. *Cure Violence* adopts a three-pronged approach that mimics an anti-epidemic strategy to stop transmission of violent behaviour. The first prong is *identification of zones of contagion*, which refers to epidemiologic mapping to localize individuals that are at high-risk of being shot or being shooters; the second prong is to *interrupt the transmission of violence*, using 'violence interrupters' (anti-violence healthcare workers) who impede the spread from person to person; and the third is *behaviour change* via, for example, community-focused events aimed at changing norms (Riemann 2019).

Through a critical discourse analysis of website content, Riemann (2019) illuminates assumptions underpinning the *Cure Violence* approach, which are illustrative of the epistemically reductive and context-stripping processes of medicalization. In the author's words,

[Cure Violence's] reliance on an epidemiological approach to violence obscures any structural, political, and sociological factors that might underpin said violence in the name of a value-free science. By conceptualizing violence as a disease that can be combated via techniques of modern epidemiology, violence becomes a biological condition alone.

(p. 151)

Riemann (2019) thus demonstrates that the medicalization of violence is connected to a neoliberal rationality where violence is understood in terms of individual pathology. This framing creates people 'at risk' who are appropriate targets for health intervention and are responsible for complying. Moreover, and significant with respect to health equity, the framing creates a racialized version of the violence 'epidemic' where "the color of susceptibility and lack of resistance is the 'non-white'". The 'visual language' of the initiative, based on the website and PowerPoint presentations prepared by Cure Violence officials, conveys that "victims, potential perpetrators, and high-risk individuals are predominantly either Hispanic or African American" (p. 152).

Biomedicalization and public health

While medicalization remains a relevant and helpful frame for conceptualizing reductive and individualistic tendencies in public health, scholars have more recently turned to theories of *biomedicalization* to better characterize the complex relationships between medicine and society. Biomedicalization signals a theoretical shift, from a normative stance focused on negative consequences of medicalization, to one inspired by the interdisciplinary field of Science & Technology Studies (STS) that is concerned with how medicine and society are co-constituted. This more recent body of theory, conceptualized by Clarke et al. (2021) as the 'next generation' of medicalization, more directly engages with the dramatic recent (since the mid-1980s) expansions of techno-scientific innovations, including computer and information sciences. For Clarke et al. (2003), the overarching analytic shift is from medical and related institutions exerting clinical and social control over particular conditions (medicalization) to an increasingly techno-scientific version of biomedicine that is capable of transforming bodies and lives.

Clarke et al. (2003, 2021) describe biomedicalization as organized around five key processes that extend into everyday experiences (see also Neresini et al. 2019):

1   Major political economic shifts under neoliberal capitalism, where biomedical research, outcomes, and services are increasingly corporatized, privatized, and multi-national;
2   A 'radical turn' towards proactive biomedical intervention in health (not just illness and injury), where health is increasingly conceived as a moral obligation and individual goal;
3   The techno-scientization of biomedicine, where things like computerized databases and genomic and molecular technologies (e.g. molecular diagnostic tests) are mobilized as 'tools' to treat and enhance the body;
4   Transformations in the production, distribution, and consumption of biomedical knowledge, in ways that reshape the boundaries between 'lay' and expert knowledge and that advance the interests of corporate biomedicine;
5   Transformations of bodies and identities, where the body is viewed as flexible and capable of being reconfigured through customized services and technologies, including those billed as 'preventive'.

Importantly, with respect to health equity concerns, scholars in this area emphasize what they call *stratified biomedicalization* or inequalities due to differential access and use of high-tech biomedicine across social axes of race, class, gender, ability, etc. (Clarke et al. 2003; Clarke et al. 2021). Stratified biomedicalization thus signals an application of *fundamental cause* theory, articulated by Link and Phelan in 1995 to describe how social factors such as class or race are 'fundamental' causes of disease because they persistently shape access to resources (i.e. money, power, connections) that can be used to avoid risks, minimize the consequences of disease, and promote health, regardless of the specific health issue or intervention (Link and Phelan 1995). Stratified biomedicalization provides a lens to illuminate contemporary manifestations of inequity, such as an excess of choice in 'boutique' biomedical technology available to some, while others continue to lack basic infrastructure and dignity. Moreover, by providing a lens to illuminate these manifestations of inequity in this 'next generation' of medicalization, stratified biomedicalization can also motivate efforts to correct injustices where, for example, structurally oppressed communities engage and mobilize science and technology (such as data) for social justice goals (Clarke et al. 2003; Clarke et al. 2021).

Since the early 2000s, processes of biomedicalization have been illuminated through in-depth empirical study. In their 2021 retrospective piece, Clarke et al. identified three overlapping areas where there has been particularly rich empirical work: (1) biomedicalization and the media; (2) biomedicalization and biomedical technologies; and (3) precision medicine and precision public health. As discussed next, recent work in these three areas illustrates the contours of biomedicalization processes and how they have shaped the field of public health.

Biomedicalization and the media in public health

Media, clearly, play a very significant role in public health as in other domains. In their editorial to a *Critical Public Health* special issue on media and public health, Henderson and Hilton (2018) emphasize that media reporting both reflects and shapes cultural ideas about public health issues; as well, it frames solutions and responsibilities in ways that are in no sense neutral or objective but rather highly social and political.

The interrelatedness of media and processes of biomedicalization is illustrated in a study by Neresini et al. (2019), which examined trends and patterns in how reporting of health, illness, and medicine was framed in UK and Italian newspapers between 1984 and 2017. Based on an analysis of publicly archived health- and medicine-related articles published in *la Repubblica* (Italy) and *The Guardian* (UK), these authors explored how public discourses serve to shape and co-constitute processes of biomedicalization. Those two newspapers were selected because they represent diverse cultural, economic, geographic, and political contexts in Europe; moreover, as 'elite' newspapers, they were thought to be particularly attentive to, including willing to question, issues of health and medicine.

Focusing on articles that explicitly referenced medical and biomedical research, technologies, and agencies, Neresini et al. (2019) noted several ways in which these media engaged with and shaped emerging biomedicalization processes including their cultural and epistemic authority. One is through the continuation of a long-standing discourse of individual responsibility, where health and well-being (not just illness and injury) are framed as matters of individual commitment to self-monitoring and self-surveillance. A second is through these newspapers' framing of biomedicine as a large techno-scientific enterprise in which emerging research fields and their technological embodiments (e.g. robotics, nanotechnologies) are strongly intertwined in media discourse about health and medicine. The authors' analysis did not reveal strong discourse around the transformation of health care in terms of growing roles of for-profit actors (i.e. the first of Clarke et al.'s five processes listed above). It thus departed from other scholarship on biomedicalization and likely reflected, according to the authors, that literature's predominant focus to date on the US context where corporatization of health care is entrenched. Overall, Neresini et al. (2019) concluded that a media analysis is a useful way to analyse general trends in the social transformation of defining, managing, and debating health and medicine, including the relatively more recent processes of biomedicalization.

Biomedicalization and biomedical technologies

A second area of important empirical work around biomedicalization and how it has shaped public health concerns biomedical technologies. Work in this area has focused on the escalation of new technologies in diverse settings – including in homes communities, and on bodies (e.g. wearable devices) where they are used as part of prevention or health promotion activities.

A paper by Carter et al. (2018) considers the biomedicalization of everyday activities, in particular the ways in which walking and cycling have been transformed by digital technologies, including wearable devices. Through a review of interdisciplinary scholarship, these authors identify several themes that illustrate the ways in which socio-technological shifts have transformed bodies, identities, communities, and relationships. One is *quantification*, meaning the expansion of digital technologies to count steps and to measure quantifiable elements of activity like distance, speed, elevation, and heart rate. Quantification, the authors note, facilitates goal setting and self-monitoring, which allow users to measure potential enhancements to their biological self. While the quantification capacity of many software applications is intended to motivate users, Carter et al. (2018) point out that their efficacy in behaviour change is debatable.

A second way in which digital technologies contribute to transforming bodies and lives is, according to Carter et al. (2018), by *reconfiguring everyday activities*. Digital technologies turn the everyday activity of walking, for example, into a health project aimed at improving biological fitness, which itself becomes defined by those aspects of walking that are discrete and countable, such as steps. In the process, however, use of those technologies can serve to diminish or relegate to the periphery other reasons for walking, like enhancing well-being by enjoying one's surroundings. With respect to cycling, the authors discuss how digital technologies reconfigure the activity by fostering competition. They do so by enabling cyclists – sometimes explicitly referred to as 'athletes' – to track and share their performance.

For both walking and cycling, interactions between technologies and bodies bring in moral elements when, for example, users feel guilty for missing a day or 'underperforming'. Carter et al. (2018) thus discuss the ways in which digital technologies for walking and cycling contribute to contemporary processes of bio-governance. They do so by creating digital citizens who are disciplined around normative expectations – around the amount of physical activity, for example – and who are willing and able to self-monitor towards those expectations. The communicative aspects of digital technologies are significant, the authors argue, with respect to transforming identities, communities, and relationships. One example of how public health and its publics are co-constituted in biomedicalization processes concerns the ability of users to share their achievements with others and to be part of a virtual community, the outcomes of which can be both positive and negative (Carter et al. 2018).

Carter et al. (2018) identify important areas for future enquiry around biomedicalization of everyday activities. One concerns scholarship, anchored in political economy, around commodification and commercial interests of biomedical technologies and corresponding equity implications, such as who gains and who loses in the expansion of digital technologies. There is also a need, the authors assert, for more work around non-users of technology. This includes 'resistors' such as cycling communities that develop their own creative commons maps in an effort to reject the commercialization of mapping software.

Precision public health

A third key area of empirical work around processes of biomedicalization and public health concerns the recent (around 2016)[2] emergence of the notion of *precision public health*.

The *precision* discourse began in medicine, where it describes efforts to tailor individual treatment strategies based on a person's clinical and genomic data. *Precision public health* signals an attempt to 'scale up' the logic of precision medicine to public health activities, including prevention and surveillance at the population level. It does so by leveraging multiple data sets and techno-sciences, often in real time, to prevent, track, and respond to communicable disease outbreaks. This includes addressing spatial inequities in health outcomes through targeted interventions (Clarke et al. 2021).

Recognizing public health's concern with social determinants of health inequities, proponents of precision public health emphasize that the approach goes beyond precision medicine's focus on clinical and genomic data to include social, environmental, and behavioural factors that contribute to differential rates of morbidity and mortality in populations. Proponents also argue that precision public health is merely an extension of epidemiology, which is concerned with the distribution and determinants of disease in populations and has long been a core aspect of public health research and practice (Clarke et al. 2021). However, considering the long-standing tensions between public health and clinical medicine and the corresponding drawbacks of attempting to scale up ideas from the latter to the former,[3] it is imperative that precision public health be considered critically. Indeed, important critical scholarship has illuminated ways in which the precision discourse and its data-driven solutions are incompatible with health equity and social justice goals.

Kenney and Mamo (2020), for example, emphasize that while precision public health techno-scientific innovations, such as using Google search data to predict influenza outbreaks, may have intuitive and popular appeal, there is little evidence that they improve health. Moreover, approaches anchored in precision discourse almost by definition tend to ignore broader social, political, and economic contexts (including those contextual factors that allow 'precision' to become attractive in the first place). Using two precision public health examples, these authors illustrate contours of biomedicalization processes and the imperative of a critical approach.

The first example, situated in global public health, is the 2011 UNAIDS Global Plan. That plan targets geographical regions in sub-Saharan Africa where HIV rates are high, and it involves treating HIV-positive pregnant women with antiretroviral therapy to prevent perinatal transmission. Kenney and Mamo (2020) effectively illustrate how *precision* is framed here as an economic necessity, because a 'blanket approach' to preventing HIV for everyone in sub-Saharan Africa is 'not practical'.[4] Consistent with neoliberal underpinnings of medicalization and biomedicalization, economic efficiency, rather than health equity, thus becomes the defining logic. Kenney and Mamo (2020) argue that the 'precision imaginary' further serves to advance a "narrative of techno-scientific progress in which smart R&D can bring humanitarian efficiency" to solve terrible global health problems. Global health initiatives, accordingly, become the domain of private philanthropic organizations, such as the Gates Foundation. Underscoring the lack of democratic accountability of a major health programme funder, the Gates Foundation, the authors argue, serves as 'neoliberal triage' by further weakening robust state responses, while leaving unquestioned and untouched the social, political, and economic systems that are the root causes of global health inequities (Kenney and Mamo 2020).

Kenney and Mamo's (2020) second example of precision public health discourse and the need to engage critically is a San Francisco, USA Cancer Initiative. 'SF CAN' was launched in 2016 with the stated aim to reduce the burden of cancer and address inequities in cancer occurrence and outcomes. The initiative is explicitly situated within 'precision population health', defined in terms of "having the data and the capability to tailor preventive interventions precisely for communities to more directly meet their needs". However, despite the initiative's prominent emphasis on equity, Kenney and Mamo (2020) point out contradictions that obstruct that goal. For example, the authors note that the slogan itself, 'SF CAN', frames cancer equity in San Francisco as attainable, despite complexities that go unacknowledged, such as increasing income inequality in the city. Moreover, the initiative's precision discourse serves to define cancer disparities as a biomedical problem that is solvable by 'big data' solutions, while omitting upstream social and structural determinants. For example, while the precision framing supports targeted interventions to reduce the risk of lung cancer from smoking in a predominantly African American neighbourhood, it would not support efforts to redress racism and income inequality because they fall outside the scope of the precision discourse.

Conclusions: opportunities to de-medicalize and re-politicize for the public's health

How and why has the field of public health, with its stated focus on upstream conditions that cause populations to be sick in the first place in a highly inequitable manner, been so powerfully shaped by reductive, individualized, and techno-solution oriented processes of medicalization and biomedicalization? Some insights may be drawn by considering public health's institutionalized history. Focusing on the American context, Yong (2021) provides a popularized account of what he calls 'public health's downfall' over the past 150 years, including how public health itself took part in it. Early 20th-century American public health, he writes, was stronger and more ambitious, drawn together by the notion that some people were more likely to be sick than others due to social conditions (see also the Introduction chapter of this volume). The solution, accordingly, was to address those conditions, including crowded housing, unsafe work, and poor sanitation. As perhaps most famously demonstrated by McKeown (see Link and Phelan 2002), broad improvements to living standards resulting from better economic conditions, rather than advances in biomedicine, demonstrably contributed to significant historical improvements in morbidity and mortality.[5]

As the 20th century progressed, however, and against the backdrop of those aggregate health improvements, the field of public health moved away from a focus on social conditions and their political aspects. A turning point, writes Yong (2021), was the late 19th-century discovery that infectious diseases were caused by microbes ('germ theory'), which "gave public health license to be less revolutionary". If the causes of disease were located in the individual body, what was the impetus to engage with much larger and more complex problems of poverty, inequality, racism, and their structural causes? Public health's shift into the laboratory created a narrow set of scientifically minded professionals, with a corresponding consolidation of professional and epistemic power. This consolidation was itself strengthened by powerful interests, including the philanthrocapitalism embodied by the Rockefeller Foundation, whose embrace of 'scientific medicine' served to legitimize the structure of capitalist society, thus contributing importantly to creating today's biomedical monopoly on health.[6]

In this context, goals and responsibilities of public health narrowed and drifted downstream to encompass data collection, diagnostic services for clinicians, disease tracing, and health education (Yong 2021). This narrow, medicalized version of public health was and continues to be perpetuated by a focus on reductive, individualized models of health protection and promotion in advanced education (college/university), including professional training in public health, especially in the North American context. Two important papers in *Critical Public Health* shed light on this medicalization of public health education, including how it manifests in the persistent omission of material like social theory (which tends to be crowded out by behavioural theory) and participatory methods (Harvey and McGladrey 2019; Yassi et al. 2019). McLaren et al. (2024b) likewise identified, focusing on Alberta, Canada, that despite stated commitments to things like equity and community, some post-secondary public health programmes are mired in an entrenched core of clinical epidemiology and biostatistics, which are taught in a highly technical manner, with other ways of thinking and knowing relegated to the periphery as optional or specialization-specific content.

If public health was once less medicalized than it is now, it can be so again. We identify two opportunities to de-medicalize public health, informed by recent critical scholarship. First is for members of public health communities, and publics, to come together to envision and work towards a *social democratic public health*. This would provide a way for public health communities to anchor in an ideological foundation other than neoliberalism, which as noted is heavily intertwined with processes of medicalization and biomedicalization. In recent critical scholarship, sociologist Sylvia Walby considers the question of social theory as it relates to public health, specifically in the context of the COVID-19 pandemic (Walby 2021; see also Speed and McLaren 2022). She identifies that, amongst the political philosophies that have been mobilized to explain the relationship between the individual and society in the context of the pandemic, social democracy has been 'curiously absent'.

This is a problem, Walby argues, for at least two reasons. First, public health and social democracy are (ostensibly) aligned. As Walby (2021) says, "Social democracy is the model of society that informs the public health project, in which 'if one is sick, we are all potentially sick' […]" (p. 24). A second reason why it is problematic to omit social democracy is because it provides a strong counter-philosophy to neoliberalism. That is, in Walby's words, "Interventionist social democratic practices can be contrasted with neoliberal policies that pursue more minimal intervention to (mistakenly) reduce damage to the economy" (p. 24). In the light of the close political economic ties between neoliberalism, medicalization, and biomedicalization, a theoretically grounded, social democratic public health represents an important opportunity indeed (see also McLaren and Mykhalovskiy 2024).

A second opportunity for de-medicalizing and re-politicizing public health involves finding ways to overcome long-standing tensions between practice (medicalized) and scholarly (critical) communities. For this, sociologist Eric Mykhalovskiy and colleagues (2019) offer important distinctions between critical social science *in*, *of*, and *with* public health, where public health refers to the medicalized version discussed in this chapter. Briefly, critical social science *in* public health describes the situation where critical scholars work within the institutional and discursive spaces of public health, such as within a university institute of public health or a public health department in a healthcare system. While this arrangement offers a way for critical scholars to contribute to applied concerns in public health, it can erode their unique analytic contributions and scholarly autonomy. In critical social science *of* public health, scholars are situated outside of public health, and the field/institution/department/profession becomes an object of inquiry; for example, scholars can illuminate reductive, individualized, decontextualized, and techno-solution oriented tendencies that are emblematic of processes of medicalization and biomedicalization. While this version of the relationship can (and has) yielded very important insights into flaws of public health practice and forms of reasoning, Mykhalovskiy et al. (2019) point out that it can turn into an entirely negative critique which points out the failings of public health but does not offer constructive alternatives.

From the point of view of working towards a de-medicalized and re-politicized public health, Mykhalovskiy et al.'s notion of critical social science *with* public health is significant as it describes a relationship that recognizes sources of difference and tension and works productively with them. While the *with* arrangement risks devolving into a superficial and uncomplicated space of shared interests, it is potentially very powerful, and indeed essential, for addressing core problems in public health such as equity, which simply cannot be solved without meaningful efforts to illuminate and question the limits placed on our thinking, knowing, and acting by processes of medicalization and biomedicalization. Critical social science *with* public health requires genuine commitment to reflexivity and ongoing engagement on both sides, which is no small challenge (Mykhalovskiy et al. 2019) but is, in our view, well worth pursuing.

Notes

1 This chapter's focus on 'medicine' refers to clinical or curative-oriented medicine, as distinct from versions of medicine that are well aligned with a broad version of public health, notably Latin American traditions of social medicine and collective health that are dedicated to theoretically robust empirical research and social and political activism to promote health and health equity through structural change (Harvey et al. 2023).

2 In the US context, a milestone was a 2016 Precision Public Health Summit co-sponsored by the University of California San Francisco (UCSF), the Obama White House, and the Gates Foundation, which posed the question, *how might precision approaches be leveraged to improve health equity?* Clarke et al. (2021) note the irony that the location of much activity around precision public health (San Francisco Bay Area and Silicon Valley) is also one where non-millionaires can barely afford to live.

3 Indeed, there are – not surprisingly – examples of the terms precision medicine and precision (public) health being used interchangeably (e.g. University of Calgary 2023), thus dismissing the very significant differences between a focus on disease at the individual level and well-being and its distribution in populations.

4 This is reminiscent of the capture of the 1978 Alma Ata Declaration's Primary Health Care agenda by vertical disease programmes, on the basis that the former was impractical and too costly. In a political economic context that set the stage for neoliberalism, it was seen as more appropriate to focus on tackling diseases with the highest prevalence, the greatest risk of mortality, and the highest possibility of control in terms of cost-effectiveness (Rifkin 2018).

5 Important subsequent work cast a critical lens on the 'McKeown thesis', pointing out that its emphasis on material living standards served to support a neoclassical economic growth and 'invisible hand' narrative that is ultimately harmful to the public's health

(Szretzer 2002). Szretzer argues that McKeown did not adequately recognize the simultaneous historical importance of other key trends such as a redistributive social philosophy, social activism and practical politics, which he notes has characterized the public health movement from its 19th-century origins.

6 For a far more in-depth analysis of the biomedical-capitalist nexus, see Brown (1979).

References

Alexander, S.A., Frohlich, K.L. and Fusco, C. (2014) '"Active play may be lots of fun, but it's certainly not frivolous": the emergence of active play as a health practice in Canadian public health', *Sociology of Health & Illness*, 36(8), pp. 1188–1204. Available at: https://doi.org/10.1111/1467-9566.12158

Brown, E.R. (1979) *Rockefeller medicine men: medicine and capitalism in America.* Berkeley: University of California Press.

Carter, S., Green, J. and Speed, E. (2018) 'Digital technologies and the biomedicalisation of everyday activities: The case of walking and cycling', *Sociology Compass*, 12(4), p. e12572. Available at: https://doi.org/10.1111/soc4.12572

Chernomas, R. and Hudson, I. (2019) 'Omission and commission in the development economics of Daron Acemoglu and Esther Duflo', *Canadian Journal of Development Studies/Revue canadienne d'études du développement*, 40(4), pp. 447–463. Available at: https://doi.org/10.1080/02255189.2019.1682976

Clark, J (2014) 'Medicalization of global health 1: has the global health agenda become too medicalized?', *Global Health Action*, 7(1), p. 23998. Available at: https://doi.org/10.3402/gha.v7.23998

Clarke, A.E. et al. (2003) 'Biomedicalization: Technoscientific transformations of health, illness, and U.S. biomedicine', *American Sociological Review*, 68(2), p. 161–194. Available at: https://doi.org/10.2307/1519765

Clarke, A.E., Jeske, M., Mamo, L. and Shim, J.K. (2021) 'Biomedicalization revisited', in W.C. Cockerham (ed.) *The Wiley Blackwell Companion to Medical Sociology.* Oxford: John Wiley & Sons, pp. 124–149.

Crawford, R. (1980) 'Healthism and the medicalization of everyday life', *International Journal of Health Services*, 10(3), pp. 365–388. Available at: https://doi.org/10.2190/3H2H-3XJN-3KAY-G9NY

Green, J. and Labonté, R.N. (eds) (2008) *Critical perspectives in public health.* London; New York: Routledge.

Hancock, T. et al. (2020) 'Opinion: there is much more to public health than COVID-19', *Healthydebate*, 15 June. Available at: https://healthydebate.ca/2020/06/topic/more-to-public-health-than-covid/

Harvey, M. and McGladrey, M. (2019) 'Explaining the origins and distribution of health and disease: an analysis of epidemiologic theory in core Master of Public Health coursework in the United States', *Critical Public Health*, 29(1), pp. 5–17. Available at: https://doi.org/10.1080/09581596.2018.1535698

Harvey, M., Piñones-Rivera, C. and Holmes, S.M. (2023) 'Structural competency, Latin American social medicine, and collective health: Exploring shared lessons through the work of Jaime Breilh', *Global Public Health*, 18(1), p. 2220023. Available at: https://doi.org/10.1080/17441692.2023.2220023

Henderson, L. and Hilton, S. (2018) 'The media and public health: where next for critical analysis?', *Critical Public Health*, 28(4), pp. 373–376. Available at: https://doi.org/10.1080/09581596.2018.1482663

Kenney, M. and Mamo, L. (2020) 'The imaginary of precision public health', *Medical Humanities*, 46(3), pp. 192–203. Available at: https://doi.org/10.1136/medhum-2018-011597

Link, B.G. and Phelan, J. (1995) 'Social conditions as fundamental causes of disease', *Journal of Health and Social Behavior*, 35, p. 80. Available at: https://doi.org/10.2307/2626958

Link, B.G. and Phelan, J.C. (2002) 'McKeown and the idea that social conditions are fundamental causes of disease', *American Journal of Public Health*, 92(5), pp. 730–732. Available at: https://doi.org/10.2105 /AJPH.92.5.730

Marelli, L., Kieslich, K. and Geiger, S. (2022) 'COVID-19 and techno-solutionism: responsibilization without contextualization?', *Critical Public Health*, 32(1), pp. 1–4. Available at: https://doi.org/10.1080/09581596.2022.2029192

McLaren, L. and Hennessy, T. (2020) 'A broader vision of public health', *The Monitor (Canadian Centre for Policy Alternatives)*, 31 December. www.policyalternatives.ca/news-research/the-monitor-january-february-2021

McLaren, L., Juzwishin, D.W.M., and Stahnisch, F.W. (2024a) 'Introduction: what is public health, and why does it matter?' In McLaren, L, Juzwishin, D.W.M., Velez Mendoza, R. (eds) *A history of public health in Alberta, 1919-2019*. Calgary, Canada: University of Calgary Press.

McLaren, L. and Mykhalovskiy, E. (2024) 'Economic policy and public health: Insights from the history of the Canadian Journal of Public Health', *Canadian Journal of Public Health*, 115(5), pp. 705–719. Available at: https://doi.org/10.17269/s41 997-024-00940-3

McLaren, L., Velez Mendoza, R., and Stahnisch, F.W. (2024b) 'Chapter 6: Public health education: power and politics in Alberta Universities' in McLaren, L, Juzwishin, D.W.M, Velez Mendoza, R. (eds) *A history of public health in Alberta, 1919-2019*. Calgary, Canada: University of Calgary Press.

Mykhalovskiy, E. *et al.* (2019) 'Critical social science *with* public health: agonism, critique and engagement', *Critical Public Health*, 29(5), pp. 522–533. Available at: https://doi.org/10.1080 /09581596.2018.1474174

Neresini, F., Crabu, S. and Di Buccio, E. (2019) 'Tracking biomedicalization in the media: public discourses on health and medicine in the UK and Italy, 1984–2017', *Social Science & Medicine*, 243, p. 112621. Available at: https://doi.org/10.1016/j.socsci med.2019.112621

Riemann, M. (2019) 'Problematizing the medicalization of violence: a critical discourse analysis of the "Cure Violence" initiative', *Critical Public Health*, 29(2), pp. 146–155. Available at: https://doi.org/10.1080 /09581596.2018.1535168

Rifkin, S.B. (2018) 'Alma Ata after 40 years: primary health care and health for all— from consensus to complexity', *BMJ Global Health*, 3(Suppl 3), p. e001188. Available at: https://doi.org/10.1136/bmjgh-2018-001188

Schrecker, T. (2022) 'What is critical about critical public health? Focus on health inequalities', *Critical Public Health*, 32(2), pp. 139–144. Available at: https://doi.org/10.1080/ 09581596.2021.1905776

Speed, E. and McLaren, L. (2022) 'Towards a theoretically grounded, social democratic public health', *Critical Public Health*, 32(5), pp. 589–591. Available at: https://doi.org/ 10.1080/09581596.2022.2119053

Szreter, S. (2002) 'Rethinking McKeown: the relationship between public health and social change', *American Journal of Public Health*, 92(5), pp. 722–725. Available at: https://doi.org/10.2105/AJPH.92.5.722

University of Calgary, Cumming School of Medicine. (2023). *Precision health: leading the future of healthcare innovation.* Available at: https://cumming.ucalgary.ca/gse/about/programs/precision-health

Valles, S.A. (2018) *Philosophy of population health: philosophy for a new public health era.* London: Routledge.

Walby, S. (2021) 'The COVID pandemic and social theory: social democracy and public health in the crisis', *European Journal of Social Theory*, 24(1), pp. 22–43. Available at: https://doi.org/10.1177/1368431020970127

Yassi, A. *et al.* (2019) 'Is public health training in Canada meeting current needs? Defrosting the paradigm freeze to respond to the post-truth era', *Critical Public Health*, 29(1), pp. 40–47. Available at: https://doi.org/10.1080/09581596.2017.1384796

Yong, E. (2021) 'How public health took part in its own downfall', *The Atlantic*, 23 October. Available at: www.theatlantic.com/health/archive/2021/10/how-public-health-took-part-its-own-downfall/620457/

4 Keeping the pressure on

Critical public health and the social determinants of health inequities

Critique of dominant approaches to understanding and promoting health – including biomedical and behavioural approaches – is an important and long-standing focus of critical public health scholarship. Critical scholars continue to be at the forefront of drawing attention to the limits of behavioural interventions in the context of structural determinants of health and of the harms of depoliticized discourses that divorce equity from its structural roots.

In this chapter, we highlight some significant contributions over the last 15 years to critical scholarship on *social determinants of health* (SDH), defined by the World Health Organization (WHO) as the quality of the conditions in which people are born, grow, live, work, and age and the wider set of social, economic, and political forces and systems that cause those conditions to be distributed in highly inequitable ways (WHO, n.d.). The first section considers the dominance of behavioural approaches to health, including the important critical concept of *lifestyle drift,* which continues to illuminate and explain how and why health behaviourism persists despite its significant drawbacks. Next, we showcase scholarship that has provided important critical nuance around the social determinants concept. To do so, we summarize work that has applied a critical lens to (1) the 2008 final report of the WHO's Commission on Social Determinants of Health (CSDH) and (2) the ensuing emphasis on intersectoral approaches to health, including a *Health in All Policies* (HiAP) approach. Finally, in the light of a growing imperative to bring together social and ecological determinants of health, the last section summarizes some important and highly prescient critical public health scholarship on ecological determinants of well-being and health equity. That final section, and indeed the whole chapter, sets the stage for our Conclusion chapter, which takes up the notion of a *well-being economy* as an alternative paradigm that centres the well-being of all people, all living things, and our planet along with the political economic structures needed to achieve such a vision.

DOI: 10.4324/9781003654650-5

The problems and unfortunate persistence of behavioural approaches to health: the imperative of a critical lens

Behavioural approaches to health are those that attribute poor health to individual lifestyle behaviours (smoking, eating poor-quality diets, drinking too much alcohol, having unsafe sex, etc.) and seek to improve health by 'helping' people to make better personal choices (the quotation marks signal questionable effectiveness and potential for harm, both of which are usually obscured in behavioural discourse). 'Helping' can involve providing information to enable people to reduce their risk, providing supports for people to change their behaviour, and creating environments that are more conducive to certain behaviours; it can also take the form of stigmatizing and shaming the undesired behaviour and those who engage in it (e.g. Bell et al. 2011).

As discussed by Chernomas and Hudson (2013), there is an important element of truth underpinning behavioural approaches – smoking and diet, for example, are associated with disease outcomes, and they contribute substantially to poor health and early death on a global scale (IHME 2024). However, as now recognized in many undergraduate social determinants textbooks (e.g. Davidson 2019) and speaking to the mainstreaming of some critical perspectives, there are very significant drawbacks of behavioural approaches, most notably that they tend to downplay or omit altogether the social and political circumstances that powerfully shape well-being and health equity. This includes but is not limited to the behavioural options available. Because they tend to be reductive and decontextualized, behavioural approaches are inherently limited in their ability to improve health at the population level, especially its inequitable distribution.

Behavioural hegemony and lifestyle drift

Despite the significant drawbacks of behavioural approaches and some general awareness of the need to recognize social circumstances, these approaches continue to dominate mainstream health discourse. Critical public health scholarship has contributed importantly to problematizing the hegemonic focus on behaviours and shedding light on how and why health behaviourism persists.

In a series of articles published in *Critical Public Health* in 2011, for example, Bell et al. (2011) consider how alcohol, tobacco, and obesity have come to be understood as dangerous problems requiring public health intervention. Bell et al. situate this framing as a predictable outcome of the dominant neoliberal political economic paradigm (see also Chapter 1 and Chapter 6 in this volume). A key element of neoliberalism's ideological intent is the liberation of individual choice, which is advanced through appealing but misleading choice-oriented narratives, which in turn serve to garner support for policy approaches like privatization and deregulation. It is not surprising, the authors argue, that in the neoliberal context, public health research, practice, and policy would come to embody that ideological orientation, manifesting as an emphasis on individual responsibility for health, an expectation of self-control over one's individual lifestyle, and attributions of failure when one does not behave in a behaviourally defined 'healthy' manner. Compounding the dominance of the individual responsibility narrative is Bell et al.'s (2011) important point that the 'danger' of health issues like alcohol, tobacco, and obesity reflects far more than ostensibly neutral statistics on their links with disease outcomes; rather, it reflects long-standing moral connotations of behaviours as 'good' or 'bad'. The resulting behavioural hegemony effectively obscures structural drivers of health problems and their highly inequitable distribution.[1]

The critical concept of *lifestyle drift* has contributed importantly to understanding the unfortunate persistence of behavioural approaches to health. Popay et al. (2010) defined *lifestyle drift* as a tendency, in policy discourse, for example, to acknowledge the need for action on upstream social determinants of health inequities only to drift downstream to ultimately focus on individual lifestyle factors. Baum and Fisher (2014) developed the concept by outlining intersecting historical, ideological, and practical reasons for why lifestyle drift occurs. A key historical factor, according to these authors, is the long-standing cultural and institutional power of clinical medicine, which has served to advance and popularize reductive biomedical and behavioural – at the expense of social and political – explanations and solutions for health problems (see also Chapter 3 in this volume). Another important historical factor contributing to lifestyle drift was the 20th-century rise of chronic diseases as major contributors to morbidity and mortality, which 'cemented' a focus on individual lifestyle behaviours and underpinned individual lifestyle-focused health education efforts (Baum and Fisher 2014).

Consistent with Bell et al. (2011), Baum and Fisher (2014) emphasize the importance to lifestyle drift of neoliberal ideology, which attributes poor health to poor 'choices' (understood in a rational, decontextualized manner) by individuals and which, coupled with dominant biomedical framing, underpins disproportionate allocation of resources to behaviourally and medically oriented research and initiatives, thus perpetuating reductive frames. Finally, Baum and Fisher (2014) argue that lifestyle drift persists due to practical factors, such as the apparent logic and simplicity of behavioural approaches as a solution to health problems, which contributes significantly to their appeal to governments. By embracing behavioural approaches, governments can appear to be 'doing something' in a way that does not require potentially contentious legislation or larger changes to the political economic status quo.

Recent critical scholarship offers theoretical nuance around how and why lifestyle drift occurs in practice. Brassolotto et al. (2014) studied health units (local public health authorities) in Ontario, Canada, with the aim of understanding why they tended to neglect the social determinants of health (SDH) in favour of health promotion approaches focused on behaviours. Across a sample of nine health units selected for their diverse engagement with SDH, these authors identified that variations in engagement reflected variations in *epistemological barriers*. Drawing from French philosopher and historian Gaston Bachelard, epistemological barriers are the worldviews and thinking patterns that must be overcome to address new problems. These intellectual hurdles, as Brassolotto et al. (2014) described them, included (1) how SDH are understood, ranging from downstream, individualized versions to upstream versions that embrace their political implications; see also Raphael (2011); (2) the role of public health units in addressing SDH, ranging from units that embraced broad engagement and advocacy roles around the SDH to units that 'stay in their lane' and consider economic structures, for example, as outside of their remit; and (3) the perceived validity of different forms of evidence and expected outcomes. For this third 'hurdle', public health units ranged from those with an allegiance to quantitative methods and discrete behavioural or disease outcomes, along with a corresponding view that the 'evidence base' for acting on SDH is limited to units that engaged more broadly with different forms of evidence and embraced process or intermediary indicators in addition to discrete downstream outcomes.

In short, and informed by these epistemological barriers, Brassolotto et al. (2014) identified that those health units that engaged the least with SDH were apprehensive or uncomfortable with the political nature of the social determinants concept. This is an important insight because it sheds light on how public health as an institution understands and acts on its stated goals to improve population well-being and health equity. The authors offer several suggestions for how those situated in formal public health structures like health units might begin to overcome these formidable barriers and strengthen the ability to engage with SDH. These include having explicit discussions within government ministries of health and public health units about the values and politics that are inherent in policy and programme decision-making; incorporating research tools that address the politics of health in meaningful ways, such as sophisticated forms of health impact assessment or application of an intersectional lens; centralizing and institutionalizing social determinants leadership, so that public health leaders' (e.g. Medical Officers of Health) personal constructions of SDH – which might be quite downstream and depoliticized – cannot take over the shape of activities; and finally, if health units have a formal responsibility for taking action on the SDH, ensuring that there is a mechanism for them to be held accountable in doing so.

In another study, Powell et al. (2017) examined how lifestyle drift played out in health promotion initiatives delivered by voluntary sector entities in the UK in the context of austerity measures implemented in the aftermath of the 2008 global financial crisis. Austerity measures (budget cuts to public services), which are a core tenet of neoliberal ideology and policy, led to increasing demands on the voluntary sector to deliver programmes that were previously part of the public sector. Those cuts were, moreover, coupled with an expectation that voluntary sector organizations would adopt business strategies that mirrored those of private sector organizations. Powell et al.'s (2017) ethnographic study was theoretically grounded in *figurative sociology*, which views systems (in this case, the voluntary sector) as networks of interdependent and dynamic relations, including relations of power. The framework thus provides a way to explore interconnections between frontline practices and dominant discourses in health promotion, such as behavioural discourses.

The study focused on health promotion initiatives in a socio-economically disadvantaged area in Northwest England ('area-based' approach) aimed at increasing physical activity, promoting healthy eating, and promoting overall well-being. Through their in-depth study, Powell et al. (2017) identified two distinct and apparently contradictory practices amongst voluntary sector providers. These practices shed light on how and why lifestyle drift occurred, despite the initiative's area-based focus on socio-economic disadvantage. On the one hand, voluntary sector providers demonstrated an empathetically informed understanding of the contexts and meanings associated with residents' use of the health promotion services. They also recognized the complexity of building understanding and trust. At the same time, however, providers tended to 'drift' into a focus on practical barriers to participation in health promotion initiatives, such as timing, location, and pricing of activities. This drift seemed to reflect an assumption that residents *should* want to participate in the initiatives. Then, when participation rates remained low even when practical barriers had been addressed, providers explained this outcome in terms of individualized, moralizing accounts of residents' attitudes, rather than considering that the whole premise of the initiative might be the problem. These individualized explanations increased in frequency as the initiative progressed, which Powell et al. (2017) point out aligns with increasing pressure for providers to meet performance targets. This study thus offers nuanced and theoretically grounded insights into lifestyle drift; it also offers applied contributions, such as the importance of reducing or removing performance-related targets from contract arrangements that appear to prompt the drift.

Behavioural approaches and blind spots in public health

Recognizing the limitations of reductive behavioural approaches to health, it is quite common in mainstream public health to see explicit (albeit sometimes vague) acknowledgement of the need to focus upstream on social determinants of health (e.g. CPHA n.d.). Despite that acknowledgement, a strong and perhaps subconscious allegiance to health behaviourism persists, and critical public health scholarship has contributed importantly to illuminating that allegiance, including how it distracts from or even obstructs meaningful efforts to redress health inequities.

One empirical illustration is a cross-sectional study by Chaufan et al. (2015) that examined the school-level (aggregate) interrelationship between active school transport (measured as the percentage of children using active forms of transport to/from school), child obesity (percentage of children meeting certain guidelines for body composition), and child poverty (percentage of children eligible for free and reduced-price meals) in California, USA. The paper is situated in the literature on child obesity, which is overwhelmingly behavioural in its orientation despite knowledge that obesity, like most other public health problems, is strongly socio-economically shaped and patterned. Chaufan et al. (2015) note that previous studies have found limited evidence for an association between active school transport and child obesity and that those studies routinely describe the lack of consistent association as 'counterintuitive'. This is, according to Chaufan et al. (2015), due to the assumption – anchored in behavioural hegemony – that active transport behaviour *should* explain child obesity.

Consistent with those previous studies, Chaufan et al. (2015) found only a weak, and in fact positive, school-level association between active school transport and child obesity (i.e. higher percentage of children engaging in active school transport, higher percentage of children with body composition consistent with obesity). Unlike other studies, however, Chaufan et al. (2015) considered and were able to explain this 'counterintuitive' finding by incorporating poverty (measured as percentage of children eligible for free or reduced-price meals) as a marker of the structural context of health behaviours. They found that schools with a higher percentage of children engaging in active school transport also had a higher percentage of children experiencing poverty and that schools with a higher percentage of children experiencing poverty also had a higher percentage of children with body composition consistent with obesity.

Chaufan et al. (2015) noted that, despite the well-established and fundamental importance of poverty to health, none of the authors of the previous studies on active school transport and child obesity interpreted their 'counterintuitive' findings from a social determinants lens. Rather, they remained committed to behavioural explanations and implications, such as making school zones safer for active transport. While such environmental changes may indeed be beneficial, Chaufan and colleagues (2015) argue that they will not eliminate nor meaningfully reduce poverty and its negative effects, pointing out that "the living conditions of the poor cannot be improved other than by addressing the institutional and political arrangements that allow poverty, and its concomitant health effects, to exist and persist" (pp. 41–42). The authors lament the 'fashionable' tendency to describe health determinants as a 'complex interplay' of various (e.g. biological, behavioural, social, cultural, environmental) factors, which dilutes the social determinants lens and serves to make poverty invisible.

Drawing parallel conclusions, but in the context of public health pedagogy, is a paper by Westbrook and Harvey (2023) that illuminated what they call 'behavioural fundamentalism' and corresponding blind spots in public health textbooks. Echoing a theme of this chapter and volume, the authors note that, despite recent and growing attention in public health to social determinants and structural approaches, a tendency persists – including in post-graduate education – to emphasize behaviours of individuals over organization of societies. To shed light on this tendency, the authors examined how the relationship amongst behaviour, society, and health is framed in commonly assigned introductory textbooks within the 'social and behavioural sciences' competency area of Master of Public Health (MPH) programmes, focusing mostly on the US context. The authors consider textbooks to be authoritative sources because, "despite their pretense to objectivity, [they] can either foreground or obscure social hierarchy, oppression, and inequitable forms of social organization" (p. 149).

Amongst the textbooks examined, Westbrook and Harvey (2023) identified several prominent tendencies in how the relationship amongst behaviour, society, and health was framed, which shed light on the insidious persistence of health behaviourism. The first was the *primacy of behaviour to health outcomes*, illustrated by opening textbook lines such as "Health behavior change is our greatest hope for reducing the burden of preventable disease and death around the world" (p. 150) or by stated major purposes of textbooks (e.g. to analyse and apply health behaviour change theories). A second key finding was textbooks' assertion that *the purpose of public health theory is to explain behaviour and inform behaviour change* or, in other words, to reduce 'public health theory' to a behavioural focus. Third, while all textbooks recognized the importance of social determinants and structural influences on health, these influences were framed as important *because* they influence health-related behaviours (and in turn health outcomes), rather than being important shapers of health in and of themselves. Finally, and consistent with Chaufan et al.'s (2015) point above about complexity, while the textbooks emphasized the need for *ecological approaches*, which recognize the need to act on various intersecting levels (individual, community, policy, etc.), the implicit or explicit purpose of these approaches is seen to be behaviour change. Overall, Westbrook and Harvey's (2023) findings illustrate a prevailing behavioural fundamentalism within mainstream public health instruction. This is problematic, they argue, because by framing the purpose of public health in terms of explaining and altering health-related behaviours, theories that seek to explain society, social hierarchy, and social structure are elided, giving the impression that such issues are beyond the scope of public health.

Critical perspectives on social determinants of health

Prompted in part by growing recognition of the limitations of behavioural approaches, there has been increasing mainstream attention to the social determinants of health in recent decades. However, while social determinants are inherently structural and upstream, the mainstreaming has meant that the concept is not always used in that way. Critical public health scholarship has contributed importantly to illuminating how and why de-politicizing of the SDH concept occurs and to 'keeping the pressure on' by advancing a version of the SDH that centres power, retaining the concept's transformative potential.

Focusing on the Canadian health research and policy context, Raphael (2011) (see also Raphael and Bryant 2023) identified numerous SDH *discourses*, or ways of talking about the SDH, that differ in terms of how social determinants and their public policy implications are understood. Discourse one, *SDH as identifying those in need of health and social services*, recognizes that those who experience adverse social determinants (poor housing, poor-quality education opportunities, etc.) have a higher likelihood of medical and social problems; the solution, accordingly, is to deliver services that meet those greater or particular needs (e.g. addressing health care needs of individuals experiencing homelessness, effectively managing chronic diseases within vulnerable communities). While these solutions are important, they are downstream and incomplete: they fail to address the reasons why people face adverse social determinants in the first place, including the inequities of power that create and perpetuate the status quo. Discourses three (*SDH as indicating the material living conditions that shape health*) and four (*SDH as indicating material living circumstances that differ as a function of group membership*) inch upstream in terms of recognizing that health is strongly shaped by the quality of living and working conditions and that those conditions are inequitably distributed across axes of class, gender, race, etc. In these discourses, however, the public policy antecedents of the inequitable distribution of social determinants are not always acknowledged, which can lead to downstream and depoliticized solutions such as clothing and food drives or literacy and counselling programmes (Raphael 2011).

Raphael's (2011) discourses six (*SDH and their distribution result from jurisdictional economic and political structures and justifying ideologies*) and seven (*SDH and their distribution result from the influence and power of those who create and benefit from social and health inequities*) are the most upstream and structural because they embrace dynamics of power. Discourse six recognizes that public policy cannot be divorced from a country's historic traditions and economic and political structures, such as white supremacy and the dominance of the market. Discourse seven incorporates the key insight that efforts to address SDH and their inequitable distribution are limited because individuals and groups *who are invested in maintaining the status quo have the power to obstruct change.* Implications of discourse seven include finding ways to educate and mobilize members of publics, through unions and other forms of collective organization, to push back against the powerful interests that result in government policy that benefits only a privileged minority and to advance alternative political economy visions (see Chapter 8, this volume). Not surprisingly, the more downstream discourses acquire far more mainstream prominence because they are unthreatening to the political status quo (Raphael 2011; Raphael and Bryant 2023).

The World Health Organization (WHO) Commission on Social Determinants of Health: critical perspectives

The 2008 release of the final report of the WHO Commission on Social Determinants of Health (CSDH) was a milestone in the mainstreaming of the SDH concept. The Commission was set up by the WHO in 2005 'in the spirit of social justice' and was tasked with marshalling the evidence on health equity, including what could be done to "close the [health equity] gap in a generation" (from the title) and to foster a global movement to do so. The report identified three overarching recommendations: (1) improve daily living conditions; (2) tackle the inequitable distribution of power, money, and resources; and (3) measure and understand the problem and assess the impact of action (CSDH 2008).

The report was, by virtually all accounts, bold and inspiring. It argued that social justice is a matter of life and death and explicitly recognized that health inequities are "not in any sense a 'natural' phenomenon but [are] the result of a toxic combination of poor social policies and programmes, unfair economic arrangements, and bad politics" (CSDH 2008, p. 1). The report's overarching recommendations left little doubt about the Commission's 'upstream' focus and its intent to avoid falling into reductive and hegemonic biomedical and behavioural ways of thinking about health and health equity.

Critical public health scholars quickly recognized the importance of the report. Baum (2008), for example, identified several substantive contributions of the work; first, it provided a 'rallying call for progressive health movements by offering a vision for a more equitable distribution of health, including the feasibility and moral importance of doing so. Second, it was, according to Baum (2008), unique amongst international commissions in its explicit focus on the role of economic policy promulgated by powerful actors such as the World Bank and the International Monetary Fund. Third, the report provided a much stronger evidence base on SDH than was previously available, including going beyond the dominant tendency to focus on diseases and behaviours. Finally, Baum (2008), who also served as a commissioner representing the People's Health Movement , a global civil society organization, noted that the Commission's engagement with civil society actors helped to address criticism of the WHO for being out of touch with communities and provided a foundation for further growth of a coherent global social movement for health.

While acknowledging the report's importance, critical scholars also raised important questions. Lee (2010), for example, discussed the global governance challenges of the report's recommendations and identified several areas where further consideration was required around effective political change strategies. One is the need to frame health equity in relation to global – as distinct from 'international' – health agendas (see also Chapter 7 in this volume) and to link health equity to other priority agendas, such as the governance of globalization in the post-2008 financial crisis context. Not doing so, Lee (2010) argues, will result in the sheer ambition of the CSDH agenda undermining its political appeal. Second while recognizing the report's impressive evidence synthesis, Lee (2010) offers the important reminder that normative differences, rather than a lack of evidence, lie at the heart of the problem of health equity: addressing health inequities is more a 'battle of values and ideas' around health equity as a goal than it is about scientific evidence.

A third critical point from Lee (2010) concerns the need for an appropriate institutional form to carry the report's recommendations forward, and it cannot be assumed that the existing multilateral system of global governance would work. Something more radical that challenges the normative frameworks underpinning contemporary multilateralism would be needed, but as Lee (2010) points out, the report is largely silent on the issue of value systems and vested interests that obstruct substantive change to dominant institutions. Indeed, the CSDH's ties to the WHO suggest a key role for that organization, but the report does not acknowledge that the WHO, in the contemporary political economic context, has less power and influence than other players in global health governance like the Gates Foundation, the World Bank, and the International Monetary Foundation. Collectively, Lee's (2010) points raise important questions around the CSDH initiative's potential for large-scale impact.

In an editorial accompanying Lee's (2010) piece, Green (2010) likewise laments the 'sheer impossibility' of the Commission's recommendations, from the perspective of the very significant theoretical, epistemological, and political divisions *within the field of public health* that would need to be overcome to achieve those recommendations. While the report's anchoring in a social justice and rights-based approach seems highly consistent with public health's commonly stated emphasis on equity, Green (2010) argues that such an approach is inherently ideological and that there are many examples of how this stance and its implications for radical social action to redistribute power are not universally held even within public health. Green's insights in that editorial speak to a key element of a critical approach in public health which was advanced in the first edition of this volume (Green and Labonté 2008), namely the imperative of looking inward (as well as outward) to reflect on our field's own internal challenges and complicity in the status quo. While Green (2010), like others, appreciates the 'uncompromising' nature of the report and its value as a rallying call, she ultimately urges caution in adopting the uncritical view that 'healthy public policy' is a win–win scenario that will benefit everyone, instead urging a critical perspective which recognizes that there will be both gains and losses for different kinds of health and for different people.

A final example of important critical perspectives on the 2008 CSDH report, which shed light on the imperative of critical perspectives on the social determinants of health more generally, is Navarro's (2009) keynote address at the 8th International Union for Health Promotion and Education European Conference, titled *What we mean by social determinants of health*. The address, with a focus on the neoliberal political economy that is dominant in and globally exported primarily by the USA, described neoliberalism's many health equity-damaging policies. These include declining public spending on public and social programmes alongside increasing public spending on military and support for private enterprises and a massive growth of both public and private investment in biomedical and genetics research (see also Chapter 3 in this volume). Navarro (2009) made a plea for stronger recognition in the SDH discourse of the importance of *class*, which he argued has almost disappeared or has been replaced by terms like 'socio-economic status', which are less collective and therefore less threatening to the social order. Class is important, Navarro (2009) argued, because neoliberalism is the ideology of the dominant classes in the global north and the global south and those class alliances are the root cause of poverty and massive inequalities (including health inequalities) within and between countries. If we are serious about the social determinants, Navarro (2009) argues that we must recognize the profound point (echoed by Raphael 2011, above) that *it is not inequalities that kill, but those who benefit from inequalities that kill.* In other words, we must engage deeply and directly with the knowledge that "disease is a social and political category imposed on people within an enormously repressive social and economic capitalist system, one that forces disease and death on the world's people" (Navarro 2009, p. 15). We take up this point, namely whether the report's recommendations were achievable without some transformations of capitalism, further in the Conclusion chapter of this volume.

Reflections on the CSDH and the need for a social determination framework

Fast forward 10 years or so, and important critical work started to emerge that reflected on the impact of the milestone Commission on Social Determinants of Health (CSDH) report in the decade following its release. Schrecker (2019), for example, considered whether, 10 years on, the Commission's work was more of a "sinking stone" or a "promise yet unrealized" (from the article's title). On the side of promise, Schrecker (2019) identified a 'conspicuous ripple' of the report in the form of an increasing number of PubMed citations about the SDH, as well as some indications of growing recognition of the political origins of health inequity. He also noted important improvements in the understanding of physiological mechanisms of health inequities (i.e. understanding how social and political dynamics of inequity and oppression get 'under the skin') and more generally a broader and richer base of evidence in support of the Commission's perspective.

However, it is hard to avoid Schrecker's (2019) "sinking stone" conclusion in that the period of the report's aftermath saw little, if any systematic efforts to address fundamental causes of health inequities. Schrecker (2019) made the extremely important yet under-recognized (in mainstream contexts) point that the report's release coincided with the hugely disruptive 2008 global financial crisis, to which dominant policy responses – including austerity – both underscored the importance of the report's recommendations *and* created very significant obstacles to achieving them.[2] These obstacles included shrinking policy space for national economic and social policy and an increasingly economically uneven distribution of political power and influence. Schrecker (2019) also identified important challenges moving forward, including limited attention to social movements which are necessary to address health inequities and the immense tensions around the assumed desirability of economic growth vis-à-vis social inequities and ecological limits.

Continuing with the 'reflections from 10 years on' theme and anchored in the persistence of dominant biomedical and behavioural approaches to health, Plamondon et al. (2020) conducted a scoping review to examine how the CSDH (2008) evidence and recommendations had been integrated into scholarly publications. Consistent with Schrecker (2019), Plamondon et al. (2020) identified that the number of publications related to SDH and health equity increased over the decade following the report's release, although the ways in which health inequities were discussed varied significantly and problematically. To analyse the publications, these authors placed each included paper on a spectrum according to how it oriented to root causes of health inequities. The spectrum ranged from less productive orientations, which included studies that *discredited*, *distracted* from, or *dismissed* root causes of health inequities, to more productive orientations, including studies that *illuminated* (made efforts to clarify or explain) root causes or that tried to *interrupt* root causes (described activities that could alter conditions that contribute to the root causes).

Overall, Plamondon et al. (2020) found limited integration of the evidence advanced by the CSDH. Only about half of the articles *problematized* health inequities by illuminating or interrupting root causes; the remainder *naturalized* health inequities by discrediting, distracting, or dismissing root causes. Of those that problematized health inequities, only a few explicitly connected health inequities to dynamics of power and privilege. On an optimistic note, articles published in the post-CSDH period and articles that directly cited the CSDH report were more likely to problematize health inequities, compared to articles in the pre-CSDH period and to articles that did not cite the report. However, there were still many articles that cited the CSDH and naturalized inequities; in other words, they misunderstood or misrepresented the report. The authors concluded that much scholarly work that purported to contribute to understanding and addressing health inequities did so in ways that conflicted with the CSDH's characterization of equity and its causes and that were inconsistent with what is required to address such inequities. This analysis raises important questions around how academic research contributes to or reinforces health inequities; at the same time, it offers opportunities to think about how research and its social, political, and economic institutions might be shifted to support more productive orientations to root causes of health inequities.

Considering trends and incisive critiques around the mainstreaming of the SDH concept, some have argued for a need to shift away from 'social determinants' language towards 'structural determinants of health' referring to the societal, economic, political, ecological, and colonial forces that cause the more proximate SDH to be inequitably distributed (e.g. CIHR-IPPH 2024; NCCDH 2022). Similar thinking, about drawbacks of 'social determinants' language, has also underpinned a proliferation of other determinants of health labelling, such as commercial determinants, ecological determinants, and political determinants, variously focusing on different structural aspects of health threat. Others in the critical space argue that despite superficial or de-politicized use of social determinants of health, the 'social' in SDH remains an important and encompassing term, so long as those using the term are thinking relationally and using theory. Muntaner and Benach (2023), for example, make this point with reference to the Weberian tradition in sociology, which distinguishes three types of *social* relations, all of which are highly pertinent to health equity: economic (i.e. relations of production, appropriation, and distribution), political (i.e. relations of power), and cultural (i.e. relations of equivalence, such as speaking the same language).

Aligning in some ways with the intent of both perspectives above is critical public health scholarship arguing for a *social determination of health* concept and paradigm, where *determination* signals that health inequities cannot be reduced to a set of discrete factors ('determinants') but rather must be understood as a series of structured processes. Anchored in Latin American traditions of 'collective health', which are themselves grounded in Marxian critiques of political economy, the social determination paradigm directly addresses important criticism of the SDH concept, namely its tendency to gloss over 'upstream' social forces that generate unhealthy social conditions; its 'truncating logic' that treats complex and interrelated phenomena as discrete and linear to the point of incorrectly representing reality; and its resulting obstruction of actions to achieve health justice by getting in the way of deeper understanding (Harvey et al. 2022).

Illustrative of the chasm between the 'social determinants' and 'social determination' paradigms, Harvey et al. (2022) note that collective health scholars perceived the emergence of 'social determinants', which occurred much later, as a reenactment of colonial relations where global north academics extracted conceptual terminology and ideas from post-colonial countries, developed them in ways that were inconsistent with or even contradicted their original meanings, and advanced them without acknowledgement of the Latin American scholars who developed them. Embracing a social determination paradigm and the profound vision of health equity that it offers requires far more than a shift in language; it demands deep, direct, and non-hierarchical engagement with the colonial origins of 'social determinants of health'. This speaks, once again, to the essential critical public health function of a critique *of* public health (see Introduction chapter), with humility to own the harms we cause as individuals and as a public health community, which may directly contradict our own stated goals as a field (Green and Labonté 2008).

Challenges of operationalizing social determinants of health in public policy: intersectoral action and the Health in All Policies approach as an illustration

Shifting to applied public health policy, we turn to a crux of the application of the SDH concept, namely that the primary determinants of population well-being and health equity lie outside of the formal health sector (e.g. ministries of health) and that coordinated action across health and non-health sectors is therefore required to achieve public health goals. A framework for realizing, such a coordinated vision is *Health in All Policies*, defined as "an approach to public policies across sectors that systematically takes into account the health implications of decisions, seeks synergies, and avoids harmful health impacts in order to improve population health and health equity" (WHO 2014).

While HiAP presents one strategy for acting on SDH, the approach – like the SDH concept itself – can be interpreted and applied in more, or less, critical ways. Indeed, consistent with *lifestyle drift* discussed above, and despite its stated focus on equity, HiAP approaches have tended to manifest in downstream, behaviour-focused goals and interventions (e.g. McLaren and Famuyide 2023). Critical public health scholarship has contributed important critical nuance and conceptual clarity around the HiAP approach, which is necessary for understanding and avoiding common and reductive explanatory traps, such as technical implementation challenges or a 'lack of political will' (Fafard et al. 2022) when the reality of implementing this approach does not match its inspiring vision.

An early scoping review by Shankardass et al. (2012) focused on government-centred intersectoral action for health equity (of which HiAP is one example) and was informed by a realist methodological lens. This review was prompted by the authors' concern that, in the context of growing interest in HiAP, literature at the time was not strongly grounded in academic analysis and showed little critical reflection. Indeed, across 128 articles describing intersectoral activities in 43 countries, the authors found that the description of the intersectoral activity was often superficial and sometimes absent, which is inconsistent with its complexity. Moreover, the vast majority of intersectoral activities described in articles reviewed by Shankardass and colleagues (2012) were 'midstream', focusing on reducing risky behaviours or exposures, or 'downstream, aiming to mitigate the inequitable impacts of up/midstream determinants such as by increasing equitable access to health care. An 'upstream' focus on structural determinants of health, including mechanisms to redistribute wealth, power, opportunities, and decision-making capacities, was essentially absent.

In a critically oriented scoping review, Chircop et al. (2015) considered the question of *how* to practise intersectoral collaboration for policy action towards health equity, which is one of the stated goals of a HiAP approach. These authors point out that intersectoral action is powerfully shaped by how the relationship between SDH and health equity is conceptualized. For example, from a neo-liberal orientation, everyone is seen as having equal access to societies' resources (including as expressed through public policy). However, this neoliberal stance obscures or negates inequities of power and privilege that underlie differences in need for or ability to use those resources, including between social groups defined by intersecting social locations, such as class, race/ethnicity, and gender. In contrast, a critical orientation takes an explicitly politicized view of health inequity as caused and perpetuated by public policies that are based on justifying ideologies that maintain power and privilege. When anchored in this observation, Chircop and colleagues argue that a key challenge (perhaps *the* key challenge) in intersectoral work is to identify and address normative assumptions of the more powerful players.

Their final sample of 64 articles was reached through a three-stage process to identify peer-reviewed scholarly papers that had a clear focus on public policy and intersectoral collaboration and that were published between approximately 1999 and 2011. Chircop et al. (2015) critically analysed those articles from the perspective of normative assumptions as noted above, and they identified several ways in which such assumptions can obstruct policy action towards health equity. First is a problematic tendency to label populations as 'vulnerable' or 'at risk' without any analysis of the social and political conditions that created that vulnerability or risk. Second, the authors note that the notion of 'intersectoral collaboration' itself in the literature is largely uncontested, suggesting a normative discourse that privileges consensus and thus silences critical voices. Third, the authors point out that the language of 'health outcomes', which often means discrete diseases, reflects and perpetuates a biomedical perspective that fails to address health equity. Fourth, a dominant focus on downstream or siloed themes, such as nutrition and mental health, suggested normative assumptions about what it meant to focus on 'determinants of health'. That is, such a focus implies that 'determinants' are specific to certain health issues, rather than consistently and fundamentally anchored in inequities in power and privilege. Finally, the authors highlighted a concentration of publications from the global north, which they argue indicated epistemic privilege and dominance. Chircop et al. (2015) concluded that these normative dimensions collectively underpin a weak political agenda for addressing health inequities and that non-critical approaches to intersectoral collaboration serve to depoliticize structures and relationships and thus undermine efforts to work towards health equity.

Based on a large mixed-methods study, Baum et al. (2014; 2017) offered critical insights into HiAP in the South Australian context, where the approach was adopted in 2007. Consistent with an emerging body of work at the intersection of public health and political science (see Fafard et al. 2022 for a recent example), Baum and colleagues emphasized the need to understand HiAP implementation not as linear or neutral but rather as a political process involving interactions between context, content, process, and power. These authors identified that a focus on *equity* varied between projects and was a contested area (Baum et al. 2014) and that some non-health sector actors equated health with hospitals and illness (Baum et al. 2017). Perhaps most significantly, the authors identified that in a neoliberal environment, 'the economy' remained the top consideration for policymakers. Indeed, one of the key factors that encouraged 'buy-in' from non-health sector public servants was finding a fit between HiAP and the dominant economic paradigm, thus raising serious questions about whether any meaningful impact is possible. Indeed, public servants were focused on working in a more coordinated and 'efficient' manner to accommodate public sector cuts; no participant questioned the cuts themselves. Baum et al. (2017) concluded that their findings supported the rather bleak recognition that neoliberalism limits "what is sayable, doable and even thinkable" (p. 14/16).

With respect to Baum et al.'s (2017) observation that some non-health sector actors demonstrated the well-known tendency to equate 'health' with hospitals and sickness, Lynch (2017) helpfully argued – based on data from 84 in-depth interviews with policymakers in four European countries (2012–2015) – that it is the 'health' part of 'health inequity' that gets in the way of meaningful efforts to redress such inequities. This occurs for two main reasons. First, the frame of 'health inequities' serves to medicalize the problem of inequity, turning what is a social and political problem into something that appears to be solvable by reductive individualized interventions within the sole remit of the health sector. Second, and most pertinent to our intersectoral discussion here, the 'health inequity' frame makes the problem seem more difficult to solve. The coherent intersectoral action (such as HiAP) required to address health inequity conflicts with the structures of most governments. It would therefore be more straightforward, Lynch argues, to focus on discrete efforts such as reducing poverty, making taxation more progressive, or implementing stronger labour market regulation. While these efforts are not politically easy, Lynch points out that they have the benefit of being relatively straightforward to imagine and of being located within single government ministries. Lynch (2017) essentially argues that while health inequity and the HiAP approach can be normative guides to public health activists, they are not necessarily useful strategic entry points to policy or political change.

A 2018 paper by Holt et al. and accompanying editorial (Rod 2018) discuss intersectoral activities within the Scandinavian context, which is commonly cited as a model for actions on upstream SDH because of its social democratic welfare regime history (Rod 2018). Holt et al. (2018) analysed documents containing recommendations for intersectoral action for health in Danish municipalities in the context of a 2007 reform that made municipalities responsible, by law, for health promotion and prevention. This included supporting the integration of health promotion within municipal services such as schools, day cares, elder care, social services, employment, and local planning. Using a neo-institutional approach, the authors explored how government-centred intersectoral action was discursively constructed in those documents by illuminating implicit expectations and contradictions.

Holt et al. (2018) identified that intersectoral action in Danish municipal contexts was discursively constructed as a 'common sense' solution, where corporate and market logics were used to present intersectoral activities as an efficient organizational response to the economic pressures of rising healthcare costs. This resulted in very high expectations (to improve the quality and efficiency of the health system) that will allegedly not require many resources. Moreover, intersectoral action's 'buzzword quality', according to the authors, conveyed a rhetorically powerful idea that is difficult to oppose, but that is also very abstract, and which obscures its inherent complexity. By advancing a corporation logic, at the expense of logics of social justice, human rights, and equity, the ambition of intersectoral action to reduce health inequities is decoupled from its political ideals (such as social justice) and presented "primarily as a technical matter which can be solved through clever organizing" (Rod 2018, p. 2). Rod (2018) makes the incisive point that intersectoral action serves a symbolic function of advancing a version of public health as a community with a collective identity and sense of purpose around SDH, which, echoing comments from Green (2010) noted above, is far from accurate.

Finally, Holt and Frohlich (2022) directly address the issue of the failure of a HiAP approach to address health inequities. They first argue for the need to distinguish between three terms that are often used interchangeably: *public health policy,* which they view as an analytical concept describing policies focused on reducing risk factors and preventing disease using individual or structural approaches; *healthy public policy,* an analytical concept based on SDH that entails upstream policies that create conditions for health, well-being, and equity; and *HiAP,* which they view as an *approach* to policymaking that involves introducing institutional arrangements to facilitate intersectoral policymaking with the goal to improve population well-being and health equity.

Using tobacco control as an example, they argue that HiAP is characterized by "confused intentionality and ambiguous directionality" (p. 273), which results in the approach being insufficient to achieve reductions in health inequities and in some cases worsening them. 'Confused intentionality' refers to public health's dual aim (intent) of (1) promoting population health and (2) reducing social inequities in health. These goals are not interchangeable, and one cannot assume that efforts to improve population-level circumstances or environments will reduce social inequities in health. 'Ambiguous directionality' refers to HiAP being described as both (1) an approach that places *health* as the main intersectoral objective and (2) a networking or collaboration strategy to advance *broader societal goals* such as sustainability and equity (conceived as determinants of health). This ambiguity is important because it carries different implications for the role and contribution of non-health sectors. The first version of HiAP (an approach with health as the main intersectoral objective) implies that non-health sectors should integrate health and health equity objectives as part of their sectoral mission and core services, while the second version (a strategy to advance broader societal goals) implies that the mission and core services of non-health sectors are recognized for their health-promoting contribution. Holt and Frohlich (2022) argue that the first description more closely resembles stated definitions of HiAP, but it is conceptually flawed because it reduces the role of non-health sectors to be implementers of health policy and neglects that their main sectoral contribution to (health) equity might be very significant. This in turn leads to the common situation in HiAP implementation where the motivation of non-health sectors to engage in the initiative is low (because their sectoral contribution is reduced or minimized). Consistent with Lynch (2017), Holt and Frohlich (2022) ultimately conclude that to meaningfully address social determinants of health equity, it is necessary to shift from a focus that centres 'health' to a focus on upstream structural drivers of inequity.

Integrating social and ecological determinants of health equity

Our final section in this chapter is inspired by a criticism that research and practice/policy around the SDH have under-emphasized or neglected *ecological* determinants such as climate change, pollution, and biodiversity loss, which collectively have massive implications for population well-being and health equity (CPHA 2015; UNFCCC 2022). This section sets the stage for a discussion in our final chapter in this volume (Chapter 8) of the notion of a *well-being economy*, briefly meaning a political economic system and paradigm that serves all people and the planet rather than the other way around. With the need for a critical perspective on this emerging idea in mind, this final section showcases important critical scholarship on ecological dimensions of well-being and health equity.

Critical public health scholarship on ecological dimensions of well-being and health equity

With climate devastation and its highly inequitable impacts no longer a distant prospect, research and scholarship on the intersection of environments, health, and (to a lesser extent) health equity have increased considerably (e.g. Potvin and Masuda 2020; The Lancet Countdown on Health and Climate Change 2023). Predating much of the recent flurry of attention is important critical scholarship on environments and health equity; here we highlight a special section of *Critical Public Health* from 2010 focused on the theme of *sustainable development, equity, and health* (Springett et al. 2010). The special section of three papers was grounded in the critical health promotion tradition, and it aligned with the 20th World Conference on Health Promotion.

The first paper, a commentary by Poland and Dooris (2010) was anchored in the observation, now much more broadly recognized, that 'progress', including improvements to aggregate population health, has come at the cost of 'staggering' damage to our environments and to most of humanity via exploitation and extraction. Moreover, the dominant solutions put forth, such as individual behaviour change or convincing businesses of the benefits of 'greening' to their bottom line, are nowhere near up to the challenge. These authors offer two important observations; the first is that few efforts to advance health or sustainability are grounded in a holistic ecological perspective, such as the *settings approach* to health promotion; and the second is that work on health and on sustainability has tended to occur in parallel rather than as integrated efforts, which reflects, in part, funding and disciplinary silos. The authors offer several principles for progressive practice at the intersection of health and sustainability. The first principle is the need to adopt an ecological 'whole system' perspective, which will facilitate moving away from a reductionist focus on single issues and linear thinking about causality. The second principle is to deepen the socio-political analysis by finding ways to connect peoples' lived experiences to those of others and to practices and structures that create and sustain dynamics of power. Overall, Poland and Dooris (2010) argue for much more radical action. They emphasize the need to avoid incrementalism as well as calls to 'balance' environmental and economic considerations when in fact they are fundamentally opposed. Presciently, these authors suggest that a 'new post-carbon society' might be the most important health promotion project of modern human history.

In the second paper, Hanlon and Carlisle (2010) made a case for reorienting public health based on immense societal challenges – such as climate change – for which the field is ill prepared. To gain insight into the challenges for public health, these authors considered the evolution of contemporary (late '00s) public discourse, policy discourse, and public health discourse around the concept of sustainability, arguing that the power of language serves to open and close various possibilities for action. In terms of *public discourse*, the authors observed threads of *alarm* (first shock and later reflective of reality); followed by *resolve* (reluctant belief); and finally *small actions* that individuals could take. The latter included varying degrees of 'techno-optimism', which the authors noted could serve to shut down discourse around the wider societal changes required. A key narrative observed in *policy discourse* was around policy action that is compatible with economic growth, underpinned by an (incorrect) belief that the two can coexist.

Hanlon and Carlisle (2010) identified two main types of *public health discourse* on sustainability: (1) the idea that knowledge from scientific evidence will inform appropriate social and policy action; and 2) repeated calls for a reorientation of public health towards deeper ecological understandings and approaches. The authors argue that these two public health discourses offer radical possibilities for action. The first possibility is for public health science to demonstrate the immense and highly unfair health implications of climate change and thus provide an 'authoritative' evidentiary foundation for radical proposals around what needs to be done (importantly, the authors note that to do so would require methodological frames that permit seeking solutions to complex and multilevel problems). The second radical possibility for public health, according to Hanlon and Carlisle (2010) is an 'ecological public health' which recognizes that natural systems, like all systems, have limits and that public health must embrace complexity, interconnectedness, and interdependence across many dimensions of life. In conclusion, these authors note that 'ecological public health' respects the historic public health task of preventing disease and promoting health, which remains relevant.

The third paper in that special section of *Critical Public Health,* by Baum and Fisher (2010), was anchored in the WHO Commission on Social Determinants of Health report (CSDH 2008) discussed above. These authors identified that, despite the fundamental importance of healthy natural environments for health and health equity, the overlap between the social determinants and climate agendas is not developed, with the CSDH report providing an example of the limited overlap. These authors identified that although the health equity consequences of climate change are very clear, those consequences tend to be framed in monetary terms like economic losses, social disruption, and lost environmental amenities. Baum and Fisher (2010) astutely pointed out that the CSDH's silence on the issue of economic growth indicates complicity with that paradigm, despite it being incompatible with its own goals. They concluded by identifying several areas where change is needed if intersecting goals of equity and sustainability are to be promoted. These include developing new indicators of economic and social development; radically restricting the dominance of transnational corporations; implementing fairer taxation and stronger tax authorities within a system of global taxation; and implementing a fairer system of global trade.

As noted in the section's editorial by Springett et al. (2010), these papers have important themes in common: recognition of the 'seriousness and immanency' of the intersecting social environmental threats; the harms embodied in social, political, and economic structures and values; and the 'profound need' for an integrated approach to social justice, equity, and broader sustainability. These themes have only become more important in the ensuing years.

Conclusion

The *social determinants of health* is an important and powerful idea in public health. It is also deceptively complex, frequently applied superficially, easily misappropriated, and overall, somewhat fraught. It thus offers a rich opportunity to illustrate the very significant contribution, or indeed the necessity, of critical perspectives. Connecting this work to the first edition of this volume (Green and Labonté 2008; see also Introduction chapter of this volume), critical scholarship on social determinants of health helps us to understand what it entails to both *look outward* and keep our focus on structural and political forces that powerfully and fundamentally shape health and its distribution, as well as to *look inward* with humility as members of public health communities for our roles in upholding those harmful systems and structures.

Notes

1 The moral connotations of behaviours and their intersection with political economy in public health have an important and interesting history. For example, as discussed by Ringen (1979) and summarized by Labonté (2024), Sir Edwin Chadwick – considered

by many to be the British 'father of public health' – sided with the miasma theory of disease contagion rather than the germ theory during the 19th century because the latter's implications for disease prevention (e.g. placing ships – the embodiment of international trade – in quarantine) were a threat to the early market society in England and the economic interests of the global merchant class with which he aligned. Moreover, an essential but rarely discussed element of the context of Chadwick's sanitary reforms is that those reforms were advanced in response to revisions to the Elizabethan-era poor laws (for which he was also responsible), which drove those living in rural poverty to urban poorhouses, where the inevitable onset of disease was attributed to "inferiority or drunken wantonness" (Labonté 2024, p. 701).

2 This can be seen as analogous to how global political economy dynamics allowed vertical or selective disease programmes, advanced by powerful people and institutions, to pre-empt comprehensive primary health care as advanced in the 1978 Alma Ata Declaration to support health for all, as noted in Chapter 3.

References

Baum, F. (2008) 'The Commission on the Social Determinants of Health: reinventing health promotion for the twenty-first century?', *Critical Public Health*, 18(4), pp. 457–466. Available at: https://doi.org/10.1080 /09581590802443612

Baum, F. and Fisher, M. (2010) 'Health equity and sustainability: extending the work of the Commission on the Social Determinants of Health', *Critical Public Health*, 20(3), pp. 311–322. Available at: https://doi.org/10.1080/09581596.2010.503266

Baum, F. and Fisher, M. (2014) 'Why behavioural health promotion endures despite its failure to reduce health inequities', *Sociology of Health & Illness*, 36(2), pp. 213–225. Available at: https://doi.org/10.1111/1467-9566.12112

Baum, F. *et al.* (2014) 'Evaluation of Health in All Policies: concept, theory and application', *Health Promotion International*, 29(suppl 1), pp. i130–i142. Available at: https://doi.org/10.1093/heapro/dau032

Baum, F. *et al.* (2017) 'Ideas, actors and institutions: lessons from South Australian Health in All Policies on what encourages other sectors' involvement', *BMC Public Health*, 17(1), p. 811. Available at: https://doi.org /10.1186/s12889-017-4821-7

Bell, K., Salmon, A. and McNaughton, D. (2011) 'Alcohol, tobacco, obesity and the new public health', *Critical Public Health*, 21(1), pp. 1–8. Available at: https://doi.org/ 10.1080/09581596.2010.530642

Brassolotto, J., Raphael, D. and Baldeo, N. (2014) 'Epistemological barriers to addressing the social determinants of health among public health professionals in Ontario, Canada: a qualitative inquiry', *Critical Public Health*, 24(3), pp. 321–336. Available at: https://doi.org/10.1080/09581596.2013.820256

Canadian Institutes of Health Research – Institute of Population and Public Health (CIHR-IPPH) (2024) *Moving upstream: structural determinants of health catalyst grant (funding opportunity)*. Ottawa: CIHR- IPPH. Available at: https://cihr-irsc.gc.ca/ e/53883.html

Canadian Public Health Association (2015) *Global change and public health: addressing the ecological determinants of health*. Discussion paper. Ottawa: CPHA. Available at: www. cpha.ca/sites/default/files /assets/policy/edh-discussion_e.pdf

Canadian Public Health Association (n.d.) *Public health: a conceptual framework (2nd edition)*. Working paper. Ottawa: CPHA. Available at: www.cpha.ca/sites/default/files/ uploads/resources/cannabis/cpha_public_health_conceptual_framework_e.pdf

Chaufan, C. *et al.* (2015) 'You can't walk or bike yourself out of the health effects of poverty: active school transport, child obesity, and blind spots in the public health literature', *Critical Public Health*, 25(1), pp. 32–47. Available at: https://doi.org/10.1080/09581 596.2014.920078

Chernomas, R. and Hudson, I. (2013) *To live and die in America: class, power, health, and healthcare*. London: Pluto Press and Black Point, Nova Scotia and Winnipeg, Manitoba: Fernwood Publishing.

Chircop, A., Bassett, R. and Taylor, E. (2015) 'Evidence on how to practice intersectoral collaboration for health equity: a scoping review', *Critical Public Health*, 25(2), pp. 178–191. Available at: https://doi.org/10.1080/09581596.2014.887831

Commission on Social Determinants of Health (CSDH) (2008) *Closing the gap in a generation: health equity through action on the social determinants of health*. Final report WHO/IER/CSDH/08.1. Geneva: Commission on Social Determinants of Health. Available at: https://iris.who.int/bitstream/handle/10665 /69832/WHO_IER_CSDH_ 08.1_eng.pdf?sequence=1

Davidson, A. (2019) *Social determinants of health: a comparative approach*. Second edition. Don Mills, Ontario, Canada: Oxford University Press.

Fafard, P. (2022) *Integrating Science and Politics for Public Health*. Cham: Springer International Publishing AG (Palgrave Studies in Public Health Policy Research Ser.).

Green, J. (2010) 'The WHO Commission on Social Determinants of Health', *Critical Public Health*, 20(1), pp. 1–4. Available at: https://doi.org/10.1080/09581590903563565

Green, J. and R.N. (eds) (2008) *Critical perspectives in public health*. London: Routledge.

Hanlon, P. and Carlisle, S. (2010) 'Re-orienting public health: rhetoric, challenges and possibilities for sustainability', *Critical Public Health*, 20(3), pp 299–309. Available at: https://doi.org/10.1080 /09581596.2010.482581

Harvey, M., Piñones-Rivera, C. and Holmes, S.M. (2022) 'Thinking with and against the Social Determinants of Health: The Latin American Social Medicine (Collective Health) Critique from Jaime Breilh', *International Journal of Health Services*, 52(4), pp. 433–441. Available at: https://doi.org/10.1177 /00207314221122657

Holt, D.H. and Frohlich, K.L. (2022) 'Moving beyond Health in All Policies: Exploring how policy could front and centre the reduction of social inequalities in health' in P. Fafard, A. Cassola, and E. De Leeuw (eds) *Integrating science and politics for public health*. Cham: Springer International Publishing, pp. 267–291. Available at: https://doi. org/10.1007/978-3-030-98985-9_12

Holt, D.H. *et al.* (2018) 'Ambiguous expectations for intersectoral action for health: a document analysis of the Danish case', *Critical Public Health*, 28(1), pp. 35–47. Available at: https://doi.org/10.1080 /09581596.2017.1288286

Institute for Health Metrics and Evaluation (IHME) (2024) *Risk factors driving the global burden of disease*. IHME. Available at: www.healthdata.org/research-analysis/library/ risk-factors-driving-global-burden-disease

Labonté, R. (2024) 'Public health can no longer fence-sit politically', *Canadian Journal of Public Health*, 115(5), pp. 701–704. Available at: https://doi.org/10.17269/s41997-024-00941-2

Lee, K. (2010) 'How do we move forward on the social determinants of health: the global governance challenges', *Critical Public Health*, 20(1), pp. 5–14. Available at: https://doi. org/10.1080/09581590903563573

Lynch, J. (2017) 'Reframing inequality? The health inequalities turn as a dangerous frame shift', *Journal of Public Health*, 39(4), pp. 653–660. Available at: https://doi.org/10.1093/ pubmed/fdw140

McLaren, L. and Famuyide, T (2023) 'What we can learn from Quebec's Health in All Policies approach', *Think Upstream*, 15 February. Available at: www.policyalternatives. ca/news-research/what-we-can-learn-from-quebecs-health-in-all-policies-approach/

Muntaner, C. and Benach, J. (2023) 'Why Social (Political, Economic, Cultural, Ecological) Determinants of Health? Part 1: *Background of a Contested Construct*', *International Journal of Social Determinants of Health and Health Services*, 53(2), pp. 117–121. Available at: https://doi.org/10.1177/27551938231152996

National Collaborating Centre for Determinants of Health (NCCDH) (2022) *Glossary of essential health equity terms*. Antigonish, NS: NCCDH, St. Francis Xavier University. Available at: https://nccdh.ca/learn /glossary.

Navarro, V. (2009) 'What we mean by Social Determinants of Health', *International Journal of Health Services*, 39(3), pp. 423–441. Available at: https://doi.org/10.2190/HS.39.3.a

Plamondon, K.M. *et al.* (2020) 'The integration of evidence from the Commission on Social Determinants of Health in the field of health equity: a scoping review', *Critical Public Health*, 30(4), pp. 415–428. Available at: https://doi.org/10.1080/09581596.2018.1551613

Poland, B. and Dooris, M. (2010) 'A green and healthy future: the settings approach to building health, equity and sustainability', *Critical Public Health*, 20(3), pp. 281–298. Available at: https://doi.org/10.1080 /09581596.2010.502931

Popay, J., Whitehead, M. and Hunter, D.J. (2010) 'Injustice is killing people on a large scale--but what is to be done about it?', *Journal of Public Health*, 32(2), pp. 148–149. Available at: https://doi.org/10.1093 /pubmed/fdq029

Potvin, L. and Masuda, J. (2020) 'Climate change: a top priority for public health', *Canadian Journal of Public Health*, 111(6), pp. 815–817. Available at: https://doi.org/10.17269/s41 997-020-00447-7

Powell, K., Thurston, M. and Bloyce, D. (2017) 'Theorising lifestyle drift in health promotion: explaining community and voluntary sector engagement practices in disadvantaged areas', *Critical Public Health*, 27(5), pp. 554–565. Available at: https://doi.org/10.1080/ 09581596.2017.1356909

Raphael, D. (2011) 'A discourse analysis of the social determinants of health', *Critical Public Health*, 21(2), pp. 221–236. Available at: https://doi.org/10.1080/09581 596.2010.485606

Raphael D. (2016) *Social determinants of health: Canadian perspectives*. Third edition. Toronto: Canadian Scholars Press.

Raphael. D. and Bryant, T. (2023) 'Socialism as the way forward: updating a discourse analysis of the social determinants of health', *Critical Public Health*, 33(4), pp. 387–394. Available at: https://doi.org/10.1080 /09581596.2023.2178387

Ringen, K. (1979) 'Edwin Chadwick, the market ideology, and sanitary reform: On the nature of the 19th-century public health movement', *International Journal of Health Services*, 9(1), pp. 107–120. Available at: https://doi.org/10.2190/LR4G-X2NK-9363-F1EC

Rod, M.H. (2018) 'The (failed) promise of intersectoral working groups and other rituals in Scandinavian public health', *Critical Public Health*, 28(1), pp. 1–3. Available at: https:// doi.org/10.1080 /09581596.2017.1396060

Schrecker, T. (2019) 'The Commission on Social Determinants of Health: Ten years on, a tale of a sinking stone, or of promise yet unrealised?', *Critical Public Health*, 29(5), pp. 610–615. Available at: https://doi.org /10.1080/09581596.2018.1516034

Shankardass, K. *et al.* (2012) 'A scoping review of intersectoral action for health equity involving governments', *International Journal of Public Health*, 57(1), pp. 25–33. Available at: https://doi.org/10.1007 /s00038-011-0302-4

Springett, J., Whitelaw, S. and Dooris, M. (2010) 'Sustainable development, equity and health–time to get radical', *Critical Public Health*, 20(3), pp. 275–280. Available at: https://doi.org/10.1080 /09581596.2010.502932

The Lancet (n.d.) 'The Lancet Countdown on Health and Climate Change'. Available at: www.thelancet.com/countdown-health-climate

United Nations Framework Convention on Climate Change (UNFCCC) (2022) 'What is the triple planetary crisis?', 13 April. Available at: https://unfccc.int/news/what-is-the-tri ple-planetary-crisis

Westbrook, M. and Harvey, M. (2023) 'Framing health, behavior, and society: a critical content analysis of public health social and behavioral science textbooks', *Critical Public Health*, 33(2), pp. 148–159. Available at: https://doi.org/10.1080/09581596.2022.2095255

World Health Organization (WHO) (n.d.) *Social determinants of health*. WHO. Available at: www.who.int/health-topics/social-determinants-of-health#tab=tab_1

World Health Organization and Ministry of Social Affairs and Health (2014) *Health in all policies: Helsinki statement. Framework for country action*. Finland: World Health Organization. Available at: https://iris.who.int/handle/10665/112636 (Accessed: 10 September 2024).

5 Beyond behaviour

Social practices and 'more than human' health

Chapter 4 highlighted critiques of the continued 'lifestyle drift' evident in public health practice and policy (Baum 2011) from the perspective of how they have sidelined action on the structural determinants of health. Behavioural interventions have also been the subject of a substantial body of critical social science scholarship for what they do, as well as what they ignore. Much of this scholarship has arisen from Foucauldian analyses of public health as an instrument of governance and disciplinary power – a particularly prevalent strand in anglophone studies (Greer and Montenegro 2023). In the introduction to *Critical Perspectives in Public Health* in 2008 (Green and Labonté, 2008), we flagged how analyses of the New Public Health, for instance, foregrounded the role of public health in creating responsibilized citizens, positioned as not only having agency to make 'healthy' choices, but also an obligation to do so (Petersen and Lupton 1996). Foucauldian analyses centred on health promotion as governance: part of a neoliberal order of governing at a distance, in which citizens internalize healthism and responsibility and discipline themselves. While this strand of scholarship continues to offer insights into the operation and social consequences of public health strategies, in the last two decades other critical approaches have begun to unsettle monolithic analyses of what health promotion and public health do in the world. These have, in part, aimed to reset the relationships between the critical social sciences and public health as both a discipline and a profession (Mykhalovskiy et al. 2019).

This chapter first briefly reviews insights from Foucauldian traditions, which continue to interrogate the role of public health within what could (at least until the 2020s) still be framed as 'neoliberal times'. Later analyses nuanced references to neoliberalism in exploring how, and in what circumstances, processes of neoliberalism have shaped the form and consequences of public health programmes. We then discuss the growing interest in theoretical traditions that open up critical analyses of public health to more normative projects, which aim towards productive and ameliorative critique, rather than simply 'denouncing' (Will 2017) the disciplining effects of public health. These approaches have drawn on diverse theories around social practice, posthumanism, and postmaterialism. Perspectives and conceptual tools from a range of social science disciplines and fields (including feminist philosophy, anthropology, geography, and Science and Technology

DOI: 10.4324/9781003654650-6

Studies (STS)) have reinvigorated social science scholarship on health promotion and public health over the last 20 years. The emphasis has shifted the object of critical enquiry away from public health as discourse and towards a new grounding in materiality, as researchers have paid close attention to what happens in practice as public health interventions roll out or new policies are implemented.

The New Public Health as governmentality

To be sure, the late 20th-century interest in public health as a plank of neoliberal governance continued into the new century, as critical scholarship engaged with changes to the forms and functions of public health practice in what were (and continue to be) in many settings periods of constrained funding (Williams and Fullager 2019). This body of work has looked at continuities and discontinuities in public health, largely in high-income anglophone countries, where the focus of prevention efforts has been on chronic disease.

Introducing a special issue on the New Public Health in 2011, Bell et al. (2011) noted some historical continuities between 19th-century health movements and the lifestyle orientations of public health in the early 21st century. Tobacco, alcohol, and obesity – the focus of their special issue – were not new objects of opprobrium and discipline: Victorian temperance movements and Protestant cultures of restraint and moderation had long targeted drinking, smoking, and overeating as moral failings. However, the New Public Health moved away from 'restraint' and moderation as the mode of intervention towards more punitive measures, particularly around smoking. Here, stigmatizing interventions and discourses brought in debates around the extent to which the ill were responsible for their own disease (and, importantly, health service costs). The critical explorations of public health responses to drugs, alcohol, and tobacco in the special issue papers touched on the often weak – or irrelevant – evidence base for the risks of behaviours in informing public health policy (such as around second-hand tobacco smoke or overweight) (Bell et al. 2011; Gard 2011), suggesting a political and ideological thrust behind much of the punitive public health discourse around behavioural risks for chronic disease. Such discourse continued to single out the most marginalized and vulnerable in society for particular opprobrium (Salmon 2011; McNaughton 2011). As Mair (2011) puts it, when behaviours (such as smoking, drinking, overeating) become reified as risks to be managed, then:

> … intervention has a tendency to become highly intrusive, selective and discriminatory and can serve to reinforce the marginalisation of the already marginalised. […] the same 'problem' populations are picked out time and time again, on behavioural grounds, for the purposes of intervention – indigenous peoples, the urban poor …
>
> (p. 130)

A theme of the papers in this special issue was the alignment of contemporary health promotion with the requirements of neoliberalism – in particular the focus on individual responsibility and choice as core to a healthy public, rather than collective action and healthy environments. Room (2011), for instance, noted that behaviouralism was an unstable solution to the contradictions between market forces that promoted alcohol consumption and the requirements for sobriety to manage modern life. However, unlike the critical responses to behaviouralism reviewed in Chapter 4, these scholars also resisted the neoliberal imperatives of 'healthism' (Crawford 1980) more broadly. LeBesco (2011), for instance, critiqued moves to reorient the focus from obese people to 'obesogenic' environments. As she notes, reconfiguring critical action away from individualistic responsibility towards action on environments leaves the dysfunctions of healthism intact: the fat body is still abject, and the moral force of prioritizing health (or its costs) above all other values persists. Instead, she argues, we need to think about alternative 'paths to well-being', including those that are explicitly resistant to biomedicalization. These might include paths that prioritize pleasure: ones that Bunton and Coveney (2011) noted were almost entirely absent in much public health discourse on drug use.

Nuancing accounts of neoliberalism

Although drawing on ideas of governmentality, and often including 'neoliberal' in their titles, few of the papers in this special issue on the New Public Health cited Foucault directly. Neither did many cite specific theoretical sources on neoliberalism. This suggests, to an extent, that ideas of both governmentality and neoliberalism had become somewhat 'black boxed' in critical public health scholarship by the beginning of the 21st century: taken for granted as frameworks for analysis of public health and health promotion policy and discourse and as a backdrop with which readers might be expected to be familiar. Indeed, some five years later, Bell and Green (2016) noted the continued routine referencing of 'neoliberalism' in public health critique, often as if this itself could 'explain' phenomena, rather than being a process in need of explanation. While acknowledging that the concept was one that could not be jettisoned, they argued that its explanatory power in critical public health scholarship might be waning, given the multiple – and indeed at times contradictory – meanings of, and consequences deemed to flow from, neoliberal health projects. As a shorthand for economic regimes (the global restructuring of capital) as well as social and cultural imperatives (a driver of governing at a distance and the marketization and individualization of health), neoliberalism was held as the explanation for all forms of public health practice and discourse. Bell and Green urged more nuance and specificity: asking not how neoliberalism was evident, but rather asking what effects the processes of neoliberalism were having in specific times and places and for whom.

Thus, Meershoek and Horstman (2016), rather than simply 'blaming' neoliberalism for a growing marketization of workplace health promotion, explored the role and consequences of public health science in commodifying occupational health in the Netherlands. Here, they argued, through providing 'evidence-based' interventions for health promotion in workplaces, such as screening questionnaires and health checks, knowledge institutes are playing a role in 'objectifying' workers, who have no voice themselves in framing demands for occupational health. Meershoek and Horstman called for a greater role for workplace unions in mobilizing to protect public health. Other analyses nuance globalizing assumptions about neoliberalism, in attending to the specificities of local manifestations. Hervik and Thurston (2016), for instance, note the complexity of Norwegian men's responses to health promotion campaigns. Although in some senses these could be framed as neoliberal, in terms of accepting personal responsibility for health, the strong welfare state in Norway and a cultural foundation of egalitarianism and collective orientation meant there was less emphasis on such issues as self-blame for ill health than found in countries such as the UK (see, e.g., Peacock et al. 2014); neither was there a rejection of the government's role in protecting health.

Unsettling the concept of 'lifestyle' diseases

The focus of many critiques of the New Public Health, and the 'lifestyle' drift of policy, whereby individual behaviours are the primary target of intervention, has been on the management of chronic diseases in high-income countries. There is often what Lindsay (2010) called a 'disconnect' between health promotion advice for healthy living and everyday life:

> Australian healthy eating and healthy drinking guidelines [...] invite us to manage our bodies in an idealised, individualised world where lifestyle change is a straightforward matter of putting knowledge into practice. Instead, we inhabit complex social worlds where food and alcohol are central to social life, and the enactment of our social identities and key social practices. Citizens do actively manage their food and alcohol consumption in an effort to be healthy, but they do so from a context where 'social wellbeing' is the primary aim.
>
> (p. 475)

At times of austerity, even the basics of public health provision for those with long-term conditions are threatened. Shaw (2018), for instance, documents the struggles of low-income patients with diabetes and hypertension in the USA to access medications at a time when bureaucratic processes were designed for cost containment by excluding as many calls on resources as possible, rather than by ensuring patients had access.

As the burden of non-communicable disease (NCD) rises globally, attention has also turned to the behavioural drift in global health, as guidelines for healthy living and programmes for disease treatment adherence developed in high-income countries are rolled out internationally. Glasgow and Schrecker (2016) discuss the "incorporation of neoliberal constructions of risk and responsibility" (p. 204) in WHO policy around chronic disease management in low- and middle-income countries to manage rapidly increasing rates of diabetes, cardiovascular diseases, and cancer across the world. Such incorporation frames chronic diseases as being related to 'lifestyle' and as preventable through modifying behaviours. Despite the inappropriateness of these approaches (in ignoring the global inequalities of trade and the limited scope of many to make healthy choices), there is a medicalization of policy, and convergence between the global north and south in approaches that resonate with neoliberal approaches to health, even if there are many examples of more upstream policy by national governments. Underpinning the export of inappropriate lifestyle advice are the universalizing tendencies of medicine, with the drive to standardize measures for diabetes, body weight, or heart rates, despite different metabolic histories and bodies (Vaughn 2019).

If there are disconnects with everyday life in the settings in which such guidelines are developed, there can be a chasm when similar advice on medication adherence and healthy living travels to other settings. Anthropology is replete with examples of the often spectacularly cruel misalignments of behaviouralist health promotion advice for chronic disease management in settings where resources are limited and contexts very different. Amy Moran-Thomas (2019), for instance, tracing the devastation wrought by diabetes in Belize, where it is a leading cause of death, points to the centuries-old histories of ecological devastation and displacement associated with colonial sugar production and trade. This is a setting of poverty, geographical marginalization, and limited health services, in which glucose testing machinery cannot be maintained, and few of the vegetables recommended on diet sheets are even available, let alone affordable. Moran-Thomas' explication of the deep-seated political causes of ill health is a devastating critique of medicalized understandings centred in the global north, and it underlines the cruel irony of characterizing diabetes as a 'lifestyle disease'.

A broader issue here is the increasingly frayed division between infectious diseases and NCDs – a division which has been at the heart of how much public health organizes itself around domains such as health promotion and health protection. As Green and Lynch (2022) note, any separation of the causes of ill health into external agents (infections, toxins) and behaviour is unsettled by the infectious disease origins of many cancers, particularly in low-income settings; by the chronicity of infectious diseases such as HIV; and by the co-location of diseases of under- and over-nutrition. Metabolic and epigenetic shifts (Landecker 2011; Vaughan 2019) have changed the ways in which bodies and environments interact first through industrialization, with its routinization of time and wakefulness, and then through post-industrial shifts to work, in which (for instance) circadian rhythms are increasingly disrupted by artificial light, shift work, and highly processed foodstuffs. The assumptions built into lifestyle approaches may be less transferable than imagined across time as well as geography. Chronic diseases are increasingly framed as 'epidemic', with what Manderson and Warren (2016) characterize as 'recursive cascades' affecting the most marginalized with multiple syndemics of chronicity caused by social and environmental conditions. There is, then, increasing pressure on simplistic behavioural models of health promotion and the dominant approaches that focus on lifestyle changes to 'modifiable risk factors'.

Resetting the relationship between critical social science and public health

Not all social science research of public health has stressed its dysfunctions or framed public health as necessarily part of neoliberal governance. Drawing on Durkheimian sociological traditions, Kevin Dew (2012) instead explored the ways in which public health practice acts as a bulwark against the excesses of capitalism, through centring phenomena such as non-market values and collective endeavour. The growing popularity of mass participation events such as 'fun runs', for instance, can be seen as arising from movements that harness solidarity and social integration in the name of public health. These Durkheimian ideas also fed into some of the work on societal responses to the COVID-19 pandemic. Mishra and Rath (2020), for instance, drawing on examples from India, discuss the forms and requirements of social solidarity when public health measures require 'social distancing' and argue that these are undermined by extreme inequalities. For Walby (2021), the challenge of the pandemic for social theory was reinserting an explicitly social democratic lens for analysing the role of public health – a lens which, she argued, underpinned the foundations of public health:

> Social democracy is the model of society that informs the public health project, in which 'if one is sick, we are all potentially sick' and in which the risks and costs associated with sickness are shared by the whole society, not only the individual who is sick.
>
> (p. 24)

Thus, for Walby, the public health response in a time of crisis was an exemplar of social democratic forms of governance that acted as a contrast to neoliberalism, rather than as agent of neoliberalism. This conceptualization of public health as social democracy, and as neoliberalism's 'other', is a counterbalance to Foucauldian critiques of science, which presume the entangling of knowledge and power and (argues Walby) imply a unified version of science. Instead, what became evident during the pandemic in many (social democratic) countries was that science was contested and multiple. Debates within science were played out in real time, in public, and (at times) scientific advice was visible as acting on policy, rather than being in the service of ideological politics. Walby's call for greater attention to social democracy, as a form of governance as well as a project, nuanced the flattening of contemporary societies as 'neoliberal', and informed calls for critical scholarship to engage more productively with what public health could do for social justice and health equity, rather than simply what it has done for governance (Speed and McLaren 2022).

However, given that anglophone critical social science scholarship, largely rooted in Foucauldian perspectives since the 1980s, had positioned public health as an instrument of governance and disciplinary power (Green and Montenegro 2023), there was little room left to engage in positive ways with public health practice. As Mykhalovskiy and colleagues (2017) put it, traditional approaches "position social science either as a conceptual resource for public health or as a source of negative critique of public health activities" (p. 522). Social sciences are either subordinate to the agenda for public health, limited in their ability to provide a unique social scientific focus, or critical, analysing public health discourse and practice as a route for theoretical novelty, not as a political project for improving health or health equity. While Foucauldian critiques have been an important strand of scholarship, analyses that simply reproduce the finding that health promotion is part of neoliberal governance absolve themselves from any obligation to advocate for different, or more productive, forms of public health practice. Seeking an alternative ethical realignment of social science with public health – rooted in what they termed 'agonism' – Mykhalovskiy and colleagues advocate for exploring "the complex, necessarily messy, but fertile space that lies in-between" (p. 523). This entails maintaining a critical disposition, but not rejecting or sidelining the endeavour of promoting health. Through seeking productive engagement with the differences between a public health orientation and a social scientific one, critical engagement can, they argue, advocate for less harmful forms of public health practice as well as developing theoretical scholarship.

For Will (2016), moving critical approaches away from simply 'denouncing' public health entailed treating its practices with care and doubt. By this she meant care about public health as an enterprise and doubt about precisely what effects public health interventions have: too often, she suggests, disciplining effects are assumed rather than demonstrated in Foucauldian critiques. Drawing on a reading of Annemarie Mol (2002; 2011) as an engagement with Foucault, Will cautions that public health in practice is unlikely to have monolithic effects, and we should instead attend to its multiplicity and differences. Interventions may, in practice, have no or few effects; they may fail to engage communities or be implemented in more conservative ways than envisaged in policy documents. A closer attention to what happens is needed, she argues, and one that takes into account the local, contingent and specific networks of people, things, and discourses that coalesce (or not) around interventions or programmes.

In this vein, for instance, Poleykett (2022) revisits a critical perspective on the 'lifestyle' drift of neoliberal global health, rejecting any easy dismissal of lifestyle health promotion for chronic disease management in Senegal as ignoring 'upstream' determinants. Although noting the inappropriateness of much behavioural health promotion advice – which assumes the existence of safe streets in which one could exercise, the availability of specific foodstuffs, and that food intake is a matter of individual choice, not household decision-making – Poleykett does not simply dismiss these efforts as failures. Instead, she attends to the ways in which people engage in complex ways with advice: women do not simply adopt or reject advice on healthy eating, for instance, but translate and negotiate this into frames that work in solidaristic or collective ways within their households. Upstream determinants, such as poverty and gendered relations, are made and reproduced at the household level, and for Poleykett, the answer is not to denounce public health efforts based on choice and agency, but rather to attend to "relational health promotion" in expanding the "latitude of social space in which people can exercise and experience agency around food" (p. 470) as well as advocating for state investments in material circumstances.

This rejection of the dualism of public health strategies and the questioning of monolithic impacts have been dominant themes in much recent scholarship in public health, which has drawn on concepts from practice theories, STS, postmaterialism, and posthumanism to make sense of the multiplicity of public health practice in terms of what it does, rather than its ideological underpinnings. What these rather disparate strands of critique have in common is a shift away from thinking about health in behavioural terms, as an outcome of individual beliefs, cognitions, and choices, and a greater attention to 'materiality' to include the non-human components of the worlds of health and health care.

The practice turn: from behaviours to practices

The 'practice turn' characterizes a shift away from researching behaviours in favour of conceptualizing what people do as 'practices'. If behaviours are properties of individuals and outcomes of cognitions, beliefs, and habits, practices are what people do in relation with others: both social and material others. To an extent, the practice turn is a correction for the disciplinary dominance of psychology in health promotion and public health practice, in particular the hegemony of various health belief and behaviour models that have become the default framing for intervention planning and evaluation. As Cohn (2014) argued, behavioural social science had become so entrenched in thinking about how to improve health, the very concept of 'behaviour' had become reified and assumed in research, rather than being an aspect of social life to explore. Further, with behaviours conceptualized as the outcomes of individual cognitions and preferences, the "social, affective, material and interrelational features of human activity are essentially eliminated" (Cohn 2014, p. 157): causal explanations then rest entirely at the micro-level. There are also, as Cohn and many others have noted, diminishing pragmatic returns from a focus on health behaviours, with evaluations increasingly failing to identify behavioural interventions as effective. While such models work well for thinking about clinical practice and issues such as individual motivations for changing behaviour, they often have little purchase on understanding the complex ways in which population-level change happens and thus offer little on the more intractable challenges for public health, such as the persistence of health inequalities.

Conversely, while structural and material critiques point to the need for social change to address enduring health inequalities, these may be perceived as offering little to practitioners on the ground in fields such as health promotion. Indeed, there has been a wealth of scholarship on the ways in which public health professionals, even when committed to action on health inequalities, hold depoliticized and individualistic models of the root causes and solutions (Brassolotto et al. 2014; Mead et al. 2022), with metaphors of 'upstream' action failing to resonate with public health actors in ways that inform policies and programmes (McMahon 2022). At a local level, practitioners struggle to consider how relational, power-infused structures can be addressed, focusing instead on targeting services at the under-served, hence the lifestyle drift documented in Chapter 4.

The promise of practice for health promotion

Practice theories are often advocated in a promissory way, with potential for bridging the gap between overly agentic and individualized models of health behaviour on the one hand and the (seemingly) abstract and difficult-to-operationalize-in-practice insights of structural analyses on the other. Thus, the promise made for social practice approaches is that they can provide pragmatic, nuanced analyses of public health challenges and ways of thinking about health improvement that are rooted in the complex ways in which health gets done. Blue et al. (2016), for instance, suggested that public health might benefit from:

> ... an alternative social-theoretical tradition: one which views the patterning of daily lives (and their implications for health) as outcomes of the coordination and synchronisation of social practices which persist over time and space, and which are reproduced and transformed by those who 'carry' them. We contend that public health policy would do better to focus on the 'lives' of social practices, treating social practices as topics of analysis and as sites of intervention in their own right.
>
> (p. 37)

Practice theories are rooted in diverse theoretical traditions. Blue and colleagues (2016) advocate an approach that draws on Reckwitz (2002) and Shove et al. (2012), to study "the patterning of daily lives (and their implications for health) as outcomes of the coordination and synchronisation of social practices which persist over time and space, and which are reproduced and transformed by those who 'carry' them" (p. 37). Enacting a practice "involves the active integration of generic 'elements', including materials/tools/infrastructures, symbolic meanings and forms of competence and practical know-how" (Blue et al. 2016, p. 41). These enactments can be sites of both disruption and reproduction; hence, they are amenable to intervention, and the study of practices can elicit productive interventions to help shift towards healthier or more equitable patterns of social practice. For Meah (2014), taking the example of domestic food safety, a key strength of a practice approach is the close attention to what people do, rather than what they say. Thus, useful evidence is more likely to come from ethnographic studies than from surveys asking for knowledge, attitudes, and beliefs. If behavioural approaches seek to understand and correct consumers' vulnerabilities to food infection risks in terms of their (faulty, lacking) knowledge and (erroneous) beliefs, a practice approach focuses instead on what people do know, and what they do, in the context of the flows of everyday life, in which several domains intersect with health. Here, embedded and embodied logics make particular practices rational in their own terms: these may or may not reflect or converge with the rationalities of food hygiene risk assessments. Rationalities of waste avoidance, for instance, may compete with those of risk reduction. While the focus on what people do is hardly new (this has long been the ethnographer's claim to useful expertise on health), reframing the object of public health research as 'practices' rather than behaviour offers a coherent set of theoretical tools to move beyond the health belief models that still dominate much public health planning.

Drawing on Bourdieu: integrating structure and agency

Other practice theories that have been applied in public health draw more on Pierre Bourdieu's *Outline of the Theory of Practice* (Bourdieu 1977), which grappled explicitly with the relationships between structures and individual subjectivity. While his body of work has traditionally been leveraged to understand how inequalities get reproduced, critical scholars have used Bourdieusian concepts to think about how practices change and what might foster healthy change. Nettleton and Green (2014), for instance, start from the challenge of the limited successes to date of health promotion interventions for increasing physical exercise, citing the division in the field between psychological approaches that focus on individual behaviour change, which inform interventions such as walking groups and 'social prescribing', and the more structural public health approaches, which are directed at changing determinants of health such as built environments in ways that encourage physical activity through making more walkable neighbourhoods or fostering everyday active transport. Robust evidence for the impact of either approach on health improvement and health equity is limited, and Nettleton and Green suggest Bourdieu's theories offer a way beyond 'theoretical dualism'.

Bourdieu's theory of practice focuses on the ways in which habitus – the routinized ways of being that we learn as tacit rules and norms – is located in particular fields, such as leisure or transport. In contrast to a psychological approach, which would conceptualize these routines as habits belonging to individuals, Bourdieu's more sociological theories incorporate relational concepts such as 'capital' to capture the different kinds of power social actors have in relation to fields and treat habitus not simply as the combined habits of individuals, but as structured by social-level relations which are internalized by individuals.

A Bourdieusian approach is dialectical, in seeking to synthesize social (relational) and individual (perceptions, cognitions) levels. Importantly, the cognitive level is therefore considered an internalization of external structures. Thus, if thinking about (for instance) increasing the amount of cycling in the population, as an intervention to foster active travel and more physical exercise, a social practice approach would explore issues such as the kinds of capital required to undertake cycling in particular fields and what kinds of tacit knowledge are embedded in the habitus of different social groups. The latter is important for practical intervention planning, as it is the taken-for-granted components of culture that make some practices 'unthinkable' for some groups, and which constitute major barriers to change. Here, proponents of these approaches argue that social science can help explicate these less easily articulated knowledges, such that interventions can be designed that are more appropriate, as they respond to what people do on the basis of taken-for-granted understandings, rather than what they say they do. Importantly, the structural elements are incorporated. Whereas behavioural models have individuals at the centre, Bourdieusian practice approaches are relational and oriented to the different levels of capital actors bring to a field. Thus, in theory, such approaches are also useful for thinking about how to design more equitable health promotion.

Both Blue et al. (2016) and Nettleton and Green (2014) proposed possible applications of social practice theory for thinking about public health interventions. The practice turn in general has informed a range of often hypothetical approaches to designing potential public health interventions: smoking (in Blue et al.'s example), health promotion for food hygiene (Meah 2014), encouraging active travel (Watson 2012; Guell et al. 2023), and risky alcohol use (Hennell et al. 2021) are some examples. Calls to address practices instead of behaviours have also begun appearing in more mainstream public health writing (see, e.g., Meier et al. 2018 on alcohol). In practice, though, such approaches remain underutilized in programme planning and evaluation, where behavioural approaches continue to dominate (see, e.g., PHE 2018).

There are, however, a few examples of social practice approaches being exploited in evaluations, in using these ideas to make sense of how, why, and in what circumstances interventions do their work, including tracing the ways in which inequities can flow from the intersections of interventions and capital. Hanckel et al. (2021), for instance, drew on Bourdieu's theories to explore the effects on school staff of a health promotion intervention to get children running for 15 minutes each day in schools. Here, they used the concept of 'hysteresis', the effect of a disconnect or time lag between field and habitus, as schools became sites of health improvement. Here, for some teachers, whose habitus was moored in a field of children's education, the shift to a field of health promotion prompted reflection, as taken-for-granted habits (such as 'teachers don't run in the playground') were made explicit by a pedagogic intervention which required teachers to engage. Exploring the reflections prompted by the new disconnect between field and habitus enabled the researchers to identify some negative outcomes of the intervention as well as positive ones, such as the ways in which it inadvertently encouraged stigmatization of body weight and reproduced class biases about food cultures. Gibson et al. (2021) also draw on Bourdieusian framings to understand how a social prescribing intervention in the UK failed to address health inequalities. Here, they focused on the particular 'capitals' needed to benefit from the intervention, including resources such as stable employment or a certain distance from necessity; for those most marginalized in society, the 'short horizons' (Warin et al. 2015) of living in a precarious and constrained present preclude attention to future term health goals.

Posthuman and postmaterialist approaches

Science and Technology Studies turns to public health

In our 2008 edition, we noted that perspectives from the Sociology of Science and Technology had begun to address public health as an area of enquiry, drawing on bodies of work such as Bruno Latour's actor–network theory and largely focusing on innovative technologies in fields such as reproduction and genetics, but that there was, at that point, little detailed analysis that took the mundane technologies of public health seriously as actors in the field (Green 2008, p. 209). That has shifted considerably over the last decades, as critical theory from STS and posthumanism has fed into research on and with public health. Will's (2020) analysis of UK public health campaigns about antimicrobial resistance (AMR), for instance, draws on STS bodies of theory on science communication to show how the imagery and format as well as texts of health promotion leaflets address the public as ignorant of antibiotics and in need of behavioural 'nudges' to prevent them from requesting inappropriate antibiotics from their doctors. This approach draws on typical Foucauldian scholarship on these texts as discourse, but Will also folds in analysis of the technologies public health actors have to 'know', such as evaluations of health promotion interventions and surveys. Here, she suggests a double role for ignorance: public responses to antibiotic prescribing are opaque and unknowable to an extent from such technologies, leaving room for behavioural economics ('nudging' behaviour) as the only possible public health response, hence health promotion campaigns have little room for reflective and thoughtful citizens or for deliberative engagements of public health and its publics.

Attending to the technologies of evidence production is a common theme in STS approaches. Horstman (2020), for instance, focuses on how different kinds of accountability are performed in practice in health promotion: what relations are made and what kinds of technologies get entangled in the doing of health. Her case study is two health promotion practices in the Netherlands: one that promoted physical activity as part of a trial and one a citizen-inspired 'Health Race' that fostered a competition between villages to become the fittest, judged by a jury of residents. While the trial had considerable scientific legitimacy, the standardized procedures, strict timelines, and professional control necessary for a trial all constrained local participation and the formation of trusting relationships. While the trial was a success in the field of public health (being held up by WHO as a 'demonstration project'), it failed to sustain health-promoting practices. The citizen-led intervention, on the other hand, was successful in that it enrolled local residents in a sustainable ongoing event and generated considerable local ownership and debate around health. However, given the need to be flexible and responsive to multiple local initiatives, the evaluation could not point to scientific success, as the goals were so diffuse. As discussed in Chapter 2, the conventional toolboxes of public health evaluation are weak for demonstrating these kinds of successes. Indeed, in Horstman's example, the organizers of the Health Race failed in their attempts to secure external funding as they could not point to the specific outcomes, or interventions, that would be fostered. Instead, the team received only a small grant for a qualitative study of participants' experiences. Horstman points to the 'collateral damage' of the unhelpful division between scientific rigour and citizen engagement, whereby successes such as those of the Health Race cannot be counted and therefore do not count, whereas the strictures of scientific accountability limit the ability to make flexible, responsive, and engaged health promotion.

Decentring the human in public health: beyond 'One Health'

Rock et al. (2014) pointed to the limitations of public health approaches that centre human health in their call for "more scholarship in public health that draws upon, interrogates, and advances debates in critical theory about non-human constituents including other animals, spaces, and technologies" (p. 337). Few of the threats to the health of people are meaningfully conceptualized as purely a 'human' problem: we live in a 'more than human' world. Infectious diseases are largely zoonotic in origin, although biomedicine separates out the management of human and animal health, and our social and physical environments shape not just risks to health, but how metabolisms work. It follows that research and action on public health needs to account for the tangled relations of human and non-human actors that make health, or health risks, in place.

Friese and Nuyts (2017) document, through a bibliometric analysis, a sharp increase in interest in non-human species in public health from 2006. However, they note that almost all this work has been conceptualized within a One Health paradigm: a vision which sought to bring together human, animal, and (later) environmental health. Other than Rock's work, they found little engagement in broader public health scholarship with the ideas of posthumanism, despite their rising prominence in the social sciences. Yet, they argue, posthuman approaches offer considerable purchase on some of the noted limitations of the One Health approach and its lack of engagement with social science. As Green (2012) noted, the One Health approach often lacked a critical edge in considering not just the interrelations of humans and animal species, but also the ways in which those relations are socially and politically made. One Health has also, in its application, been locked into anthropocentrism: Kamenshchikova et al.'s (2021) review of policy documents found an overriding framing of threats to human health, with the veterinary and environmental sectors positioned as responsible for dealing with those.

Posthuman approaches go further than One Health in acknowledging that flourishing has to be a "multi-species endeavour" (Rock 2017, p. 321). In addition to simply including non-human species in models of health, posthumanism decentres the human as the primary concern and critiques assumptions that we are (or should be) embedded in the humanism of both post-enlightenment social science and public health as an endeavour. Post-enlightenment social sciences in public health have too often taken divisions (human/non-human; material/social; male/female) as if they were categories in the world, rather than contingent, multiple accomplishments. Rock et al. (2014) reviewed some of the (disparate) traditions that have contributed to this decentring of the human, which have built on and critiqued the scholarship of Foucault and Bourdieu, drawing on the insights of STS on the material as well as social constructions of science, on feminist postmaterialism and on developments in geography and elsewhere on 'non-representational theory' (Thrift 1996).

Coin and Lynch (2017), in a special issue devoted to posthuman approaches, noted that the range of perspectives encompassed by the term is vast – and that not all scholars working on related areas would label their approach as posthuman. Non-human phenomena have always been central to public health: toxins, pump handles, mosquitoes, sewers, and air are all major characters in the stories public health tells of its origins and its contemporary challenges. Cohn and Lynch argue that what is different about a posthuman approach is that these are treated as actors with potential agency, rather than just as objects that the social acts upon. Countering the objection that attributing non-humans with agency simply "risks the wrath" of critics, Cohn and Lynch (2017) suggest some advantages of doing this:

> At one level, the point is simple; to present accounts of humans and non-humans in common ways, so that we don't inadvertently assume from the outset that one is more important, or has more influence, than any other [...] a posthumanism conviction [is] not to automatically accord humans with an exceptional status, and instead find ways to present non-human elements with equivalence. [...] we should not assume from the outset that humans will always be the central focus of our attention, but they instead constitute only one category amongst a range of different kinds of actors.
>
> (pp. 285–286)

This perspective brings symmetry to analysis, whereby the human actor is not assumed to be at the centre, and the researcher is forced to account for the role of the social, rather than take it for granted. For Cohn and Lynch, this is not simply a theoretical point, but one that offers potential insights for public health. First, methodologically, it provides the possibility of reframing problems, bringing fresh ways of considering solutions to intractable challenges. Addressing AMR, for instance, can be rethought as a challenge of 'microbial relations' rather than one of human behaviour. Second, in terms of ontology, shifting the human from the centre of our models of health and well-being might open up new, relational ways of thinking about health that are more attuned to complex ways in which health is maintained or damaged and suggest new spaces for intervention.

New materialisms

Posthuman and postmaterial approaches share a focus on how things are made with social constructionist accounts, but their focus is on 'enactment': how heterogeneous networks of (human, material, digital) actors, through practices, bring things into being. Thus, entities (diseases, health risks, digital data) are not stable, nor are they the outcomes of purely social interaction. Rather, they are inherently unstable, liable to come apart, and be differently enacted within different networks. Fox (2016) characterized the diverse strands of theory that take 'matter' seriously, including those looking at affect, relationality, and posthuman philosophy as the 'new materialisms'. He notes that these "encompass a dizzying array of perspectives, from actor–network theory, biophilosophy, feminist and queer theory, non-representational theory, post-humanism, quantum physics and Spinozist affect theory" (p. 68), but suggests common threads in a rejection of top-down concepts of power in favour of a focus on the micropolitics of how power makes things possible or constrains. Thus, the focus is on what happens on the ground, in the local and contingent relations that are made when health promotion unfolds in specific spaces.

Dennis's (2017) account of the 'injecting event' is a good example of how this work has been applied. She critiques the humanism of many harm reduction approaches in drug use, instead turning her focus on the material as well as human elements of using drugs, in aiming to "use the concepts of 'contingency' and 'care' to rebuild optimism in a harm reduction that no longer requires a bounded human and instead strives to attune to these human and nonhuman processes, to reconfigure bodies in 'healthier' ways" (p. 337). Thus, the aim is not simply to critique harm reduction (or other approaches to drug use) as perpetuating a neoliberal discourse of the rational, health seeking individual, but rather to expand our understanding of what is happening when drugs are injected to rethink what it might mean to intervene in ways that foster health. This account draws on a range of theoretical inspirations that are common in posthuman approaches, including Karen Barad's (2007) concept of 'intra-action', which captures the ways in which two actors are not interacting as separate beings, but co-constituting each other relationally, and Gilles Deleuze (1990), whose 'relational ontology' assumed no pre-existing forms and structures, but rather focused on their 'becoming' through process and on 'events' in which such becomings were actualized. There is also a political and ethical dimension: drawing on Braidotti (2013), whose project was to think more productively with 'difference', Dennis is interested in an ethics of expanded intra-relations that include matter as well as people. Dennis therefore focuses on the 'becomings-with' drugs that emerge, including those related to pleasure, and on the ways in which they were blocked or enabled by, for instance, different opiate alternatives, or external materialities such as the opening hours of services or availability of housing.

Promise, but as yet unrealized?

Critical scholarship continues to document and critique the 'lifestyle drift' (Baum and Fisher 2014) that has proved so resilient as a framework in public health (Baum and Fisher 2014; Williams and Fullager 2019; Warin and Zivkovic 2019). Despite decades of evidence around both the empirical limitations of this approach (which does little to address health inequalities) and its ideological basis (as a plank of neoliberal governance), across many settings, behavioural biases appear to have a centrifugal force for public health policy, practice, and evaluation. Yet, for critical scholars, there are also diminishing returns in simply pointing to this tendency. Seeking to reinvigorate productive critique over the last two decades, scholars from diverse perspectives have engaged in more granular ways with public health practice, addressing what happens when health promotion does get rolled out or when practitioners do intervene in the world. This body of work has often aimed to sidestep the conventional alignments of social sciences as either subservient 'in' public health, or as critical 'of' public health (Mykhalovskiy and Weir 2019) through an explicit aim of providing critique attuned to the range of both actualized effects and alternative possibilities that roll out from public health programmes.

However, the pessimist might argue that – at least to date – this scholarship has failed to live up to its promise. While offering new questions and perspectives for the analysis of public health practices (see, e.g., Lupton 2019; Fox and Klein 2020) and a wealth of academic outputs with nuanced descriptions of how health practices get done, it has perhaps under-delivered in terms of practical suggestions or evidence of uptake. At times, the conclusions from sophisticated analyses drawing on postmaterialist theory and feminist philosophy have little more purchase than any other style of detailed qualitative research. Pragmatically, psychological behavioural models continue to dominate planning and evaluation (PHE 2018; Will 2020), and researchers continue to document the drift to behaviouralism on the front line (Warin and Zivkovic 2019). There are few examples of practice theories, posthuman, or postmaterialist framings informing the design of health promotion or being integrated fully in evaluation. The nuanced findings of much posthuman research, which resist simplistic causal explanations, or holistic claims around effects, might in theory resonate with practitioners, but offer little over and above their own experiential knowledge of the effects of programmes in practice. Typically, those at the front line of delivery and planning are well aware of complexity and contingency, yet have to act in the light of uncertainty. Faithful descriptions of their work and the work of the publics they interact with, or speculations on how things might be other, may be satisfying at the level of description and thought experiment, but perhaps less fruitful for informing the next steps in settings where action is constrained. Further, with behaviouralism still entrenched at the level of international and national policy, securing funds to plan, implement, and evaluate interventions from other perspectives is likely to be challenging.

Yet, more optimistically, the impacts of social science insights tend to be more diffuse and longer term, and the more 'agnostic' stance vis-à-vis public health has the potential to open up more productive engagements between qualitative research and public health practice. Certainly, there are signs that concepts such as social practice are being taken up. Blue et al.'s (2016) paper on social practice approaches for public health has been well cited, including in mainstream public health journals, and there is some modest evidence of more social models of health practices being taken up in intervention planning, despite the continued dominance of behaviour change theory (see, e.g., McQuoid et al. 2023 on smoking cessation interventions). Given the crisis in methodologies for evaluative public health that we documented in Chapter 2, there is considerable space for approaches that do offer nuanced analysis of what interventions do, beyond the narrow effects that are prioritized in trials.

Conclusion

Critical scholarship has continued to document the inappropriate dominance of behaviouralism in public health policy and practice, but, over the last two decades, this has increasingly drawn on a wider range of theoretical underpinnings than the Foucauldian analyses that dominated critical public health in the late twentieth century. Taking inspiration from feminist philosophy, STS, posthumanism, and postmaterialist approaches, a large body of empirical research on health promotion and public health has made three key contributions. First, it has generated interest in a set of conceptual tools that provide ways of thinking about health practices that go 'beyond behaviour' in attending to the ways in which health (and illness) are 'done' within relations that include not just other people, but also non-human agents. Second, this recent scholarship has reinvigorated what had become rather tired assumptions about the role of public health in neoliberalism and its mono-lithic impacts. Third, and related, there has been a recalibration of the relation-ship of social science and public health, such that critical studies can be political, and ethically engaged, but from the perspective of productive critique, rather than condemnation.

References

Barad, K.M. (2007) *Meeting the universe halfway: quantum physics and the entanglement of matter and meaning*. Durham: Duke University Press.

Baum, F. (2011) 'From Norm to Eric: avoiding lifestyle drift in Australian health policy', *Australian and New Zealand Journal of Public Health*, 35(5), pp. 404–406. Available at: https://doi.org/10.1111 /j.1753-6405.2011.00756.x

Baum, F. and Fisher, M. (2014) 'Why behavioural health promotion endures despite its failure to reduce health inequities', *Sociology of Health & Illness*, 36(2), pp. 213–225. Available at: https://doi.org/10.1111 /1467-9566.12112

Bell, K., Salmon, A. and McNaughton, D. (2011) 'Alcohol, tobacco, obesity and the new public health', *Critical Public Health*, 21(1), pp. 1–8. Available at: https://doi.org/10.1080/ 09581596.2010.530642;www.tandfonline.com/doi/abs/10.1080/09581596.2010.530642

Blue, S. et al. (2016) 'Theories of practice and public health: understanding (un)healthy practices', *Critical Public Health*, 26(1), pp. 36–50. Available at: https://doi.org/10.1080/ 09581596.2014.980396;www.tandfonline.com/doi/full/10.1080/09581596.2014.980396

Bourdieu, P. (1977) *Outline of a theory of practice*. Translated by R. Nice. Cambridge: Cambridge University Press (Cambridge studies in social and cultural anthro-pology, 16). Available at: https://doi.org/10.1017 /CBO9780511812507

Braidotti, R. (2013) *The posthuman*. Cambridge, UK; Malden, MA, USA: Polity Press.

Brassolotto, J., Raphael, D. and Baldeo, N. (2014) 'Epistemological barriers to addressing the social determinants of health among public health professionals in Ontario, Canada: a qualitative inquiry', *Critical Public Health*, 24(3), pp. 321–336. Available at: 10.1080/ 09581596.2013.820256; www.tandfonline.com/doi/abs/10.1080/09581596.2010.530644

Bunton, R. and Coveney, J. (2011) 'Drugs' pleasures', *Critical Public Health*, 21(1), pp. 9–23. Available at: https://doi.org/10.1080/09581596.2010.530644

Cohn, S. (2014) 'From health behaviours to health practices: an introduction', *Sociology of Health & Illness*, 36(2), pp. 157–162. Available at: https://doi.org/10.1111/ 1467-9566.12140

Cohn, S. and Lynch, R. (2017) 'Posthuman perspectives: relevance for a global public health', *Critical Public Health*, 27(3), pp. 285–292. Available at: https://doi.org/10.1080/ 09581596.2017.1302557

Crawford, R. (1980) 'Healthism and the medicalization of everyday life', *International Journal of Health Services*, 10(3), pp. 365–388. Available at: https://doi.org/10.2190/3h2h-3xjn-3kay-g9ny

Deleuze, G. (1990) *The logic of sense*. Edited by C.V. Boundas. Translated by M. Lester and C.J. Stivale. New York: Columbia University Press.

Dennis, F. (2018) 'The injecting "event": harm reduction beyond the human', in S. Cohn and R. Lynch (eds) *Posthumanism and Public Health*. 1st edn. Routledge, pp. 53–65. Available at: https://doi.org/10.4324 /9781315102184-6

Dew, K. (2012) *The cult and science of public health: a sociological investigation*. New York: Berghahn Books.

Fox, N.J. (2016) 'Health sociology from post-structuralism to the new materialisms', *Health: An Interdisciplinary Journal for the Social Study of Health, Illness and Medicine*, 20(1), pp. 62–74. Available at: https://journals.sagepub.com/doi/10.1177/1363459315615393

Fox, N. J., & Klein, E. (2020). The micropolitics of behavioural interventions: a new materialist analysis. *BioSocieties*, 15(2), pp. 226–244.

Gard, M. (2011) 'Truth, belief and the cultural politics of obesity scholarship and public health policy', *Critical Public Health*, 21(1), pp. 37–48. Available at: https://doi.org/10.1080/09581596.2010.529421

Gibson, K., Pollard, T.M. and Moffatt, S. (2021) 'Social prescribing and classed inequality: a journey of upward health mobility?', *Social Science & Medicine*, 280, p. 114037. Available at: https://doi.org/10.1016 /j.socscimed.2021.114037

Glasgow, S. and Schrecker, T. (2016) 'The double burden of neoliberalism? Noncommunicable disease policies and the global political economy of risk', *Health & Place*, 39, pp. 204–211. Available at: https://doi.org/10.1016/j.healthplace.2016.04.003

Green, J. (2008) 'Introduction: Edgy spaces: technology, the environment and public health' in J. Green and R. Labonté (eds) *Critical perspectives in public health*. London: Routledge.

Green, J. (2012) '"One health, one medicine" and critical public health', *Critical Public Health*, 22(4), pp. 377–381. Available at: https://doi.org/10.1080/09581596.2012.723395;www.tandfonline.com/doi/full/10.1080/09581596.2012.723395Che

Green, J. and Lynch, R. (2022) 'Rethinking chronicity: public health and the problem of temporality', *Critical Public Health*, 32(4), pp. 433–437. Available at: www.tandfonline.com/doi/full/10.1080/09581596.2012.723395

Green, J. and Montenegro, C. (2023) 'Sociologies of public health and health promotion', in A. Petersen (ed.) *Handbook on the Sociology of Health and Medicine*. Cheltenham, Glos: Edward Elgar Publishing, pp. 308–323. Available at: https://doi.org/10.4337/9781839104756.00029

Guell, C., Ogilvie, D. and Green, J. (2023) 'Changing mobility practices. Can meta-ethnography inform transferable and policy-relevant theory?', *Social Science & Medicine*, 337, 116253. www.sciencedirect.com/science/article/pii/S027795362300610X?via%3Dihub

Hanckel, B., Milton, S. and Green, J. (2021) 'Unruly bodies: resistance, (in)action and hysteresis in a public health intervention', *Social Theory & Health*, 19(3), pp. 263–281. Available at: https://doi.org/10.1057 /s41285-020-00143-z

Hennell, K., Piacentini, M. and Limmer, M. (2021) '"Go hard or go home": a social practice theory approach to young people's "risky" alcohol consumption practices', *Critical Public Health*, 31(1), pp. 66–76. Available at: https://doi.org/10.1080/09581596.2019.1686460

Hervik, S.E.K. and Thurston, M. (2016) '"It's not the government's responsibility to get me out running 10 km four times a week" – Norwegian men's understandings of responsibility for health', *Critical Public Health*, 26(3), pp. 333–342. Available at: https://doi.org/10.1080/09581596.2015.1096914

Horstman, K. (2020) 'Performing health promotion: an analysis of epistemic and political technologies of accountability', *Critical Public Health*, 30(5), pp. 589–600. Available at: Https://doi.org/10.1080 /09581596.2019.1654600

Kamenshchikova, A. *et al.* (2021) 'Anthropocentric framings of One Health: an analysis of international antimicrobial resistance policy documents', *Critical Public Health*, 31(3), pp. 306–315. Available at: https://doi.org/10.1080/09581596.2019.1684442

Landecker, H. (2011) 'Food as exposure: nutritional epigenetics and the new metabolism', *BioSocieties*, 6(2), pp. 167–194. Available at: https://doi.org/10.1057/biosoc.2011.1

LeBesco, K. (2011) 'Neoliberalism, public health, and the moral perils of fatness', *Critical Public Health*, 21(2), pp. 153–164. Available at: https://doi.org/10.1080/09581596.2010.529422

Lindsay, J. (2010) 'Healthy living guidelines and the disconnect with everyday life', *Critical Public Health*, 20(4), pp. 475–487. Available at: https://doi.org/10.1080/09581596.2010.505977

Lupton, D. (2019) 'Toward a more-than-human analysis of digital health: inspirations from feminist new materialism', *Qualitative Health Research*, 29(14), pp. 1998–2009. Available at: https://doi.org/10.1177 /1049732319833368

Mair, M. (2011) 'Deconstructing behavioural classifications: tobacco control, "professional vision" and the tobacco user as a site of governmental intervention', *Critical Public Health*, 21(2), pp. 129–140. Available at: https://doi.org/10.1080/09581596.2010.529423

Manderson, L. and Warren, N. (2016) '"Just one thing after another": recursive cascades and chronic conditions', *Medical Anthropology Quarterly*, 30(4), pp. 479–497. Available at: https://doi.org/10.1111 /maq.12277

McMahon, N.E. (2022) 'Working "upstream" to reduce social inequalities in health: a qualitative study of how partners in an applied health research collaboration interpret the metaphor', *Critical Public Health*, 32(5), pp. 654–664. Available at: https://doi.org/10.1080/09581596.2021.1931663

McNaughton, D. (2011) 'From the womb to the tomb: obesity and maternal responsibility', *Critical Public Health*, 21(2), pp. 179–190. Available at: https://doi.org/10.1080/09581 596.2010.523680

McQuoid, J. *et al.* (2023) 'Tobacco cessation and prevention interventions for sexual and/or gender minority-identified people and the theories that underpin them: a scoping review', *Nicotine and Tobacco Research*, 25(6), pp. 1065–1073. Available at: https://doi.org/10.1093/ntr/ntad018

Mead R., Thurston, M. and Bloyce, D. (2022) 'From public issues to personal troubles: individualising social inequalities in health within local public health partnerships', *Critical Public Health*, 32(2), pp. 168–180. Available at: https://doi.org/10.1080/09581596.2020.1763916

Meah, A. (2014) 'Still blaming the consumer? Geographies of responsibility in domestic food safety practices', *Critical Public Health*, 24(1), pp. 88–103. Available at: https://doi.org/10.1080 /09581596.2013.791387

Meershoek, A. and Horstman, K. (2016) 'Creating a market in workplace health promotion: the performative role of public health sciences and technologies', *Critical Public Health*, 26(3), pp. 269–280. Available at: https://doi.org/10.1080/09581596.2015.1015489

Meier, P.S., Warde, A. and Holmes, J. (2018) 'All drinking is not equal: how a social practice theory lens could enhance public health research on alcohol and other health behaviours', *Addiction*, 113(2), pp. 206–213. Available at: https://doi.org/10.1111/add.13895

Mishra, C. and Rath, N. (2020) 'Social solidarity during a pandemic: through and beyond Durkheimian lens', *Social Sciences & Humanities Open*, 2(1), p. 100079. Available at: https://doi.org/10.1016 /j.ssaho.2020.100079

Mol, A. (2002) *The body multiple: ontology in medical practice*. Durham, North Carolina: Duke University Press. Available at: https://doi.org/10.1215/9780822384151.

Mol, A. (2011) *The logic of care: health and the problem of patient choice*. London: Routledge.

Moran-Thomas, A. (2019) *Traveling with sugar: chronicles of a global epidemic*. Oakland, California: University of California Press.

Mykhalovskiy, E. *et al.* (2019) 'Critical social science *with* public health: agonism, critique and engagement', *Critical Public Health*, 29(5), pp. 522–533. Available at: https://doi.org/10.1080 /09581596.2018.1474174

Nettleton, S. and Green, J. (2014) 'Thinking about changing mobility practices: how a social practice approach can help', *Sociology of Health & Illness*, 36(2), pp. 239–251. Available at: https://doi.org/10.1111 /1467-9566.12101

Peacock, M., Bissell, P. and Owen, J. (2014) 'Dependency denied: Health inequalities in the neo-liberal era', *Social Science & Medicine*, 118, pp. 173–180. Available at: https://doi.org/10.1016/j.socscimed.2014.08.006

Petersen, A. and Lupton, D. (1996) *The New Public Health: health and self in the age of risk*. London Kingdom: Sage.

Poleykett, B. (2022) 'Collective eating and the management of chronic disease in Dakar: translating and enacting dietary advice', *Critical Public Health*, 32(4), pp. 462–471. Available at: https://doi.org/10.1080 /09581596.2021.1898545

Public Health England (2018) *Improving people's health: applying behavioural and social sciences to improve population health and wellbeing in England*. Guidance 2018478. Public Health England. Available at: https://assets.publishing.service.gov.uk/media/5bb21dd2e5274a3e0d7af9e0/Improving_Peoples_Health_Behavioural_Strategy.pdf

Reckwitz, A. (2002) 'Toward a theory of social practices: a development in culturalist theorizing', *European Journal of Social Theory*, 5(2), pp. 243–263. Available at: https://doi.org/10.1177 /13684310222225432

Rock, M. J. (2017). Who or what is 'the public' in critical public health? Reflections on posthumanism and anthropological engagements with One Health. *Critical Public Health*, 27(3), 314–324

Rock, M.J., Degeling, C. and Blue, G. (2014) 'Toward stronger theory in critical public health: insights from debates surrounding posthumanism', *Critical Public Health*, 24(3), pp. 337–348. Available at: https://doi.org /10.1080/09581596.2013.827325

Room, R. (2011) 'Addiction and personal responsibility as solutions to the contradictions of neoliberal consumerism', *Critical Public Health*, 21(2), pp. 141–151. Available at: https://doi.org/10.1080 /09581596.2010.529424

Salmon, A. (2011) 'Aboriginal mothering, FASD prevention and the contestations of neo-liberal citizenship', *Critical Public Health*, 21(2), pp. 165–178. Available at: https://doi.org/10.1080/09581596.2010.530643

Shaw, S.J. (2018) 'The pharmaceutical regulation of chronic disease among the U.S. urban poor: an ethnographic study of accountability', *Critical Public Health*, 28(2), pp. 165–176. Available at: https://doi.org/10.1080/09581596.2017.1332338

Shove, E., Pantzar, M. and Watson, M. (2012) *The dynamics of social practice: everyday life and how it changes*. Los Angeles: SAGE.

Speed, E. and McLaren, L. (2022) 'Towards a theoretically grounded, social democratic public health', *Critical Public Health*, 32(5), pp. 589–591. Available at: https://doi.org/10.1080/09581596.2022.2119053; www.tandfonline.com/doi/full/10.1080/09581596.2022 2119053

Thrift, N.J. (1996) *Spatial formations*. London.

Vaughan, M. (2019) 'Conceptualising metabolic disorder in Southern Africa: Biology, history and global health', *BioSocieties*, 14(1), pp. 123–142. Available at: https://doi.org/10.1057/s41292-018-0122-3

Walby, S. (2021). 'The COVID pandemic and social theory: social democracy and public health in the crisis', *European Journal of Social Theory*, 24(1), pp. 22–43.

Warin, M. and Zivkovic, T. (2019) 'Romantic complexity and the slippery slope to lifestyle drift', in Warin, M. and Zivkovic, T., *Fatness, obesity, and disadvantage in the Australian suburbs*. Cham: Springer International Publishing, pp. 91–121. Available at: https://doi.org/10.1007/978-3-030-01009-6_4

Warin, M. *et al.* (2015) 'Short horizons and obesity futures: disjunctures between public health interventions and everyday temporalities', *Social Science & Medicine*, 128, pp. 309–315. Available at: https://doi.org /10.1016/j.socscimed.2015.01.026

Watson, M. (2012) 'How theories of practice can inform transition to a decarbonised transport system', *Journal of Transport Geography*, 24, pp. 488–496. Available at: https://doi.org/10.1016 /j.jtrangeo.2012.04.002

Will, C.M. (2017) 'On difference and doubt as tools for critical engagement with public health', *Critical Public Health*, 27(3), pp. 293–302. Available at: https://doi.org/10.1080/09581596.2016.1239815

Will, C.M. (2020) 'The problem and the productivity of ignorance: public health campaigns on antibiotic stewardship', *The Sociological Review*, 68(1), pp. 55–76. Available at: https://doi.org/10.1177 /0038026119887330

Williams, O. and Fullagar, S. (2019) 'Lifestyle drift and the phenomenon of "citizen shift" in contemporary UK health policy', *Sociology of Health & Illness*, 41(1), pp. 20–35. Available at: https://doi.org/10.1111/1467-9566.12783

6 Beyond the state

The health perils of neoliberal globalization

Public health has long had to pay some attention to disease threats originating beyond national borders, most notably infectious diseases. Since the early 19th century, at least, public health efforts to prevent diseases conflicted with mercantile interests in trade and commerce (Labonté and Ruckert 2019). This chapter provides an update of this historic tension. It begins by discussing the conceptual shift from international health to global health, drawing on critiques of how economic and political processes at a global scale are affecting opportunities for health. It then turns its attention to 'globalization', a newly minted term that describes societal processes of much longer lineage. It focuses on the post-1980s widespread adoption of neoliberal economics and its disequalizing impacts on health outcomes and its instantiation in public and policy discourse where it functions (in postmodern terms) as a form of 'governmentality'. The chapter moves on to 'austerity', the persisting and pervasive neoliberal economic tenet premised on disciplining excess public spending in order to sustain private wealth accumulation. The chapter's final two sections assess: firstly, the health implications of 'free' trade and investment treaties, which are the legal entrenchments of neoliberal theory's emphasis on market primacy and deregulation; and secondly, how these new international rules manifest in the global diffusion of unhealthy commodities or what has become known as the commercial or corporate determinants of health.

From international to global health and back again

The first critical issue in interrogating global health is defining what is meant by the term. It is a relatively new concept, with *PubMed* archives suggesting that it only emerged as a citable term around 1980. Until then, as Labonté and Torgerson (2008) noted in the first edition of this book (Green and Labonté 2008), "researchers, development agencies and non-governmental organizations (NGOs) mobilized around 'international health' issues: the greater burden of disease faced by poor groups in poor countries" (p. 163). The older concept of international health still outperformed its global variant in public health literature until 2013, when global health stole the lead and has been in citable first place since (Labonté and Ruckert 2019). One reason for this shift in nomenclature is that 'international

DOI: 10.4324/9781003654650-7

health' though still commonly used, is tainted with its association with colonial authorities and corporate philanthropies that imposed disease control measures on poorer countries primarily to protect their expat and border-residing citizens or to advance their geopolitical and economic interests (Labonté and Ruckert 2019).

Recent global health scholarship discriminates between three related concepts: public health (bounded within nations), international health (concern for health of people in other nations), and global health (focusing on issues that transcend national boundaries, the COVID-19 pandemic being a recent exemplar) (Koplan et al. 2009). The delineations are not always neat, and a critical social science appreciation of the malleability of social constructs would have us be more concerned with how these terms are explicated and operationalized than with how they are definitionally circumscribed. Nonetheless, the concept of global health has enjoyed a rapid ascendance over the past decade, with global health programmes sprouting up in universities worldwide. This growth has not gone without critique, notably that such programmes often manifest the same international health "asymmetries in … who designs and who receives global health interventions", reproducing "colonial cleavages that shaped the historical interaction between 'the west and the rest''' (Montenegro et al. 2020, p. 127). Global health students, researchers, and practitioners remain predominantly based in high-income countries (HIC), while their work (their practice laboratories) is more commonly situated in LIC with lagging health indices.[1]

While there is a decolonizing pushback against this anachronistic legacy, the legacy persists, often manifesting as little more than fly-by data gathering in low-income countries (LICs) by high-income country (HIC) researchers with analysis, publication, and academic credits accruing northwards. This practice, although now under more critical scrutiny and likely diminishing (e.g. many global health funders encourage or require local research or implementation partners), nonetheless "consolidated a certain global distribution of expertise (in the 'north') and need (in the 'south')" in which teaching global health is something best done "in certain places (like London or New York) but not in others (like Santiago or Abuja)" (Montenegro et al. 2020, pp. 127–128). Writing from the vantage of the global south, Montenegro and colleagues (2020) identified two key strategies to overcoming this academic hegemony: first, global health materials (texts, curricula) must be polylingual to break the restricting monopoly of English, and second, biomedical predominance must be challenged by greater recognition of "the perspectives of sociology, anthropology, historiography, and political science" to permit much stronger "focus on local conditions and sociocultural foundations of health and illness" (Montenegro et al. 2020, p. 128).

In a similar vein, Kingori and Greets (2019) regard global health as still being hostage to the "tenacious idea … that institutions, politics, and ideologies from the Global South fall short of those from the North; the Global South[2] can at best imitate, mimic, or copy those associated with the North" (2019, p. 382). An example of what the authors call 'pseudo global health' (where 'pseudo' means the indeterminate space between what is considered 'real' and 'fake') is the widespread assumption that generic (copied) medicines produced in the south are likely to be substandard or counterfeit, while their patented originals in the north are authentic (Hodges 2019). Although there are egregious cases of falsified drugs emanating from plants in India or China (Lambert 2019), there is no shortage of similar or parallel cases involving Big Pharma firms based in the USA, UK, and European Union (EU) (Wikipedia 2023; Light et al. 2013). North or south, what drives such corruption is the pursuit of profit. Another example of 'pseudo global health', also discussed in Chapter 1 of this volume, is the assumption that academic journals originating in the south are predatory, marketed to researchers in LICs as affordable open-access options to advance their careers but wholly lacking in the rigour (authenticity) of highly ranked journals published in the north (Allman 2019). Some academic journals do meet these criteria (many of us are daily bombarded by these in our academic email accounts), but not all. And it is the north's high-ranked journals, with their costly article processing charges (APCs) and reliance on publicly funded research, researchers, and peer-reviewed processes, that routinely achieve predatory profit margins exceeding 30 per cent (Lange 2022; see also the Introduction chapter of this volume).

Faking global health

A variant of the 'pseudo' problem is what Erikson (2019) described provocatively (and deliberately) as 'faking global health', in which dominant economic rationalities – such as 'return on investment' – skew public health interventions into activities with an *appearance* of global health but with little improvement in the conditions that create disproportionate disease risks (emphasis in original). The case study was the 2014–2016 Ebola outbreak in Sierra Leone; the three global health ideas found to be 'faking it' were health security, health innovation, and health financing.

First, prior to the 2014 Ebola outbreak, Sierra Leone on paper demonstrated good health security, complying with all the obligations of the World Health Organization's (WHO's) International Health Regulations.[3] However, as described by Erikson:

> These requirements assure the world that health surveillance systems are in place to detect disease threats. The *appearance* of disease preparedness was good enough for the international community, until it wasn't.
>
> (p. 509)

Sierra Leone, a LIC, is not alone in this; the two most highly rated countries for pandemic preparedness prior to COVID-19, at least on paper, were the USA and the UK, which subsequently ranked first and third amongst HICs for having the worst pandemic outcomes (Worldometer 2023). As Erikson's commentary laments, global health actors are "creating environments where everyday systems to care for the documents are usually more demanding than those caring for people" (p. 511).

Second, health innovation, echoing the north/south critique, is embedded primarily in HIC institutions eager to attract "investor financing". In Sierra Leone, this innovation showed up as new digital technologies (big data tools) that, by tracking people and disease, claimed to be capable of creating effective containment models. As Erikson noted:

> The *appearance* of contagion-control innovation was enough to justify the attempted cooptation of West African telecommunications companies' time, data, and attention during a pandemic. Computational epidemiologists insisted their containment model would work, until it didn't.
>
> (p. 509)

As with other health technology innovations, 'faking it' has to do with assumptions about transferability; in this instance, an assumption that a data analytic for an endemic disease (malaria) could work for a pandemic outbreak (Ebola) and in a context where cell phones are unlinked to specific individuals and network coverage is spotty.

Third, health financing suffers a similar critique, with the West Africa Ebola outbreak appearing just as global health was in "the throes of massive experimentation in humanitarian aid and global health funding", including "impact bonds, blended finance, angel investing, and [new] finance facilities" (p. 509). As described again by Erikson:

> In global health, financial innovation has come to mean the creating and popularising of capital market instruments [which] *appear* to be easy remedies to the increasing reticence of wealthy countries to give money to poor countries for emergency response or assist in the cultivation of health systems.
>
> (p. 509)

The West Africa Ebola outbreak gave rise to a new financial innovation, the WB's Pandemic Emergency Financing Facility. Investors could buy 'pandemic bonds' which, in the absence of a declared pandemic, would reward them with 13% annual interest. They could lose some of their investment if a pandemic was declared, but the terms for making such a declaration were highly restrictive and would see the release of new financing too late to assist in outbreak containment (Jonas 2019). When the Facility was scrapped in 2020 because of these criticisms, the conditions to release $200 million of its $320 million in bonds had finally been met. Bond investors had already been paid $100 million in interest, which, with the $120 million in bonds that would be returned to them, meant they had still enjoyed a $20 million return on investment (Hodgson 2020).[4]

From global health to globalization

While 'faking' or 'pseudo' global health scholarship yields important critical insights, where it perhaps falls short is in accounting for why some countries are poor and more disease-burdened than others; that is, what drives global disparities in the first place? There are hints of an answer in an oft-cited definition of global health that describes its emphasis as "transnational health issues, *determinants*, and solutions" (emphasis added) (Koplan et al. 2009, p. 1995). Another concept that emerged in the scholarly literature in the 1980s is globalization, which provided a frame for elaborating on these determinants. Like global health, globalization had earlier iterations such as imperialism (the conquests, rise, and fall of pre-modern empires) and colonization (the 'discovery' and claiming of 'new' lands by Western European powers). Like global health, it has had many definitional suitors, summed up by Labonté and Torgerson (2008) in this book's first edition as "processes by which nations, businesses, and people are becoming more connected and inter-dependent via increased economic integration and communication exchange, cultural diffusion [...] and travel" (2008, p. 162). Their emphasis on processes is important: globalization is less an end state than "an unstoppable dynamic embedded in industrialisation and the rise of nation-states, a 'World Systems' logic in which capitalism from its very inception was inherently globalising" (Labonté 2008, p. 138). As Larkin (2008) explained:

... contemporary processes of globalisation are constituting themselves within a context already marked by inequalities carried over from the earlier colonial phase, and it is relative to these patterns of inequality that people and states in the poorer countries must currently engage with globalisation. The importance of these unequal relations can be seen in the ways in which communities and states in the poorer regions have become caught up in Western-driven development agendas which appear to be out of their control and have had serious negative consequences for health.

(p. 154)

The same year this book's first edition was published (Green and Labonté 2008) the WHO's Commission on the Social Determinants of Health released its final report, with its provocative claim that "social injustice is killing people on a grand scale" as the result of "the unequal distribution of power, income, goods, and services, globally and nationally" (Commission on the Social Determinants of Health 2008).[5] The evidence-base substantiating this claim came from the work of nine knowledge networks, one of which focused on globalization as a "determinant of the social determinants of health". This network contrasted its analytical positioning with those that offer "simply descriptive accounts of globalization that do not attempt to identify connections among superficially unrelated elements or to assign causal priority to a specific set of mechanisms" arguing instead that "since the early 1980s and the rise of neoliberalism, economic globalization has been the driving force" (Labonté and Schrecker 2007, p. 5).

Despite the evidence for this conclusion and continuing research and scholarship in this domain, the economic (neoliberal capitalist) paradigm that has defined the past four decades of globalization has been largely ignored in public/global health teaching and research. This, at least, is White's finding from a 2012 study of public health schools in the USA. As one of the faculty interviewees in this study noted:

> Everyone gives lip service to the notion that this thing called globalization is happening ... but very few people are investigating globalization as a root cause directly.
>
> (p. 288)

When economic globalization does appear on global health curricula, it is usually optional, not core. One reason White gives for this absence is that public health faculty "are not well prepared or comfortable teaching this topic" (p. 288) given its demand for some fluency in political economy, but it thereby creates a vicious cycle of ill-prepared and uncomfortable future faculty and a "public health [that] is not living up to its rich history of proactively tackling political and economic structures shaping health" (p. 291). There is some online evidence of new global health programmes more explicitly addressing economic globalization as a determinant of health, but, generally, most programmes remain grounded in biomedicine with only limited social or political science expertise.

Neoliberalism and the rise of contemporary globalization

Globalization, at least in the meaning of increased global economic integration that White (2012) found to be missing from most global health programmes, has nonetheless been declared dead or dying for many years. The hyper-globalization of the past four decades may be in retreat, as it has been since the 2008 global financial crisis and the recessionary decline in growth in high- and upper-middle-income countries. As a recent commentary put it, "in GDP terms at least, we may have reached peak [economic] globalization" (Labonté et al. 2022, p. 2/4). This does not mean that we will enter a period of 'deglobalization' in which, outside of unilaterally declared trade wars, countries revert to the extreme protectionism that ended an earlier period of (largely European) economic integration and that led to both world wars (Labonté and Ruckert 2019). It does mean, however, that the dynamics underpinning globalization are in flux, including the neoliberal economic orthodoxy that gained geopolitical prominence in the 1980s (see also the Conclusion chapter of this volume).

Neoliberalism is an extension of Western liberalism that first arose in the transition from feudalism to capitalism during the 17th and 18th centuries. The divine right of kings was replaced by the notion of individuals enjoying natural rights and the idea that governments are legitimate only to the degree that they receive the consent of the governed. Liberal thought also embedded itself in a laissez-faire economics that emphasized how markets' 'invisible hand' allows the self-interested actions of individuals to benefit all: the oft-cited example is the baker maximizing his own economic well-being by making and selling the bread needed by others (the male possessive adjective is deliberate; it would be a few centuries before women were also regarded as individuals with rights). In contrast to the 'free market' narrative, early proponents of market economics, such as Adam Smith, nonetheless recognized that markets needed government intervention to avoid extremes of poverty and to ensure social harmony by providing tax-subsidized public infrastructure, goods, and education (Labonté and Ruckert 2019). Nonetheless, economic liberalism of varying deference to governments' role has been a mainstay of Western capitalism ever since.

The architects of 'neo'-liberalism's more extreme form began their intellectual redesign shortly after the Second World War, but it was not until the 1970s that a confluence of financial crises ('stagflation' and a declining rate of profit in the advanced economies, a new oil cartel creating fossil fuel price shocks, and a sovereign debt crisis in the developing world) combined with conservative politics (the election of Thatcher in the UK and Reagan in the USA) allowed neoliberalism to displace the more regulatory and redistributive Keynesian economics that had dominated the post-war period.[6] Neoliberalism's basic tenets are attributed to one of its founders, Friedrich Hayek, who distilled classical liberalism to a belief that free markets, sovereign individuals, free trade, strong property rights, and minimal government interference were essential to human well-being.[7] Economics was best left to individual choices in an unencumbered market.

Neoliberalism was essentially absent from critical public health discourse and analysis at the time of the book's first edition but has mushroomed since. Bell and Green (2016) in a keyword search of recent *Critical Public Health* articles found 93 references to the term, often used adjectively as in 'neoliberal this' or 'neoliberal that', chiding somewhat this neoliberal appending to most things public health and health promotion without describing what the term is meant to convey and rarely focusing on its economic underpinnings. There are differing ways in which social science use of the concept has been parsed, but, at base, neoliberalism can be seen as having two dominant meanings: first, as a macroeconomic system aligned with most of Hayek's key tenets, including an ideologically infused 'rolling back' and 'rolling out' of state formations, albeit with the depth of policy and programme compliance varying by country; and second, as a totalizing 'rationality' in the Foucauldian sense, "linked less to economic dogmas or class projects than to specific mechanisms of government, and recognizable modes of creating subjects" (Ferguson 2010), often described as 'governmentality'. In both instances neoliberalism functions as a hegemonic discourse, a way of circumscribing what is "sayable, doable, and even thinkable" (Rushton and Williams 2012, p. 149) in much the same manner that Thatcherism in the UK spawned the acronym TINA to justify her conservative/neoliberal policies: 'There Is No Alternative'.

Neoliberal macroeconomics

Of the first, macroeconomic, usage, Labonté (2012) posited a model of neoliberal policy passing through three identifiable phases:

1   The structural adjustment programmes (SAPs) of the 1980s and 1990s, where neoliberal conditionalities attached to developing country loans or grants from the IMF and WB led to a 'roll back' of government welfare state spending;

2 The financialization of the global economy from the late 1990s onwards, a 'rollout' of largely unregulated global banks and financial instruments (derivatives) allowing speculators to earn millions or billions simply by betting on financial markets;

3 Austerity, the voluntary or imposed fiscal retrenchment, manifesting as dramatic cuts to public sector supports and services, that followed massive government spending to bail out the global economy following the 2008 financial crisis, itself precipitated by unregulated global finance.

Much of the critical global public health writing since the beginning of the present millennium focused on structural adjustment and its suite of policies nominally argued to be essential to stimulate economic growth but primarily intended to stabilize the global financial system. These include privatizing state assets to pay off international loans, reducing subsidies for food and housing, imposing user fees for basic services, de-regulating to enable private sector-led growth, lowering corporate or marginal tax rates or offering tax holidays to attract foreign investment, and rapidly opening economies to global markets through trade and financial liberalization (Labonté and Ruckert 2019; Larkin 2008). SAPs failed to create the promised growth (UNDESA 2006) but, despite encouragement that health spending be somewhat protected from cuts, succeeded in socio-health impacts that were singularly negative and hardest on women, those living in poverty, children, and rural communities (SAPRIN 2002).

The financialization of the global economy marked a different iteration of neoliberalism's underlying axiomata. As Ruckert and Labonté (2012) point out, the global integration and deregulation of liberalized financial markets, repeal of laws separating commercial from investment banking, and suffusion of new digital technologies generated massive asset bubbles that created one small crisis after another before culminating in the 2008 global meltdown. De Vogli and Owusu (2014) place the greatest blame on two key US government deregulatory decisions:

> In 1999, the US Congress ... repealed the 1933 Glass-Steagall Act, which was developed by Roosevelt in response to the 1929 crash as a means of controlling risky speculations in the banking sector. By dismantling the 'wall' separating investment banks from commercial banks and insurance companies, this ... marked a watershed in the proliferation of the financial products that caused the last global crisis. The rescinding of the Glass-Steagall Act allowed large commercial lenders to underwrite and trade very profitable new speculative instruments and relaxed the requirements for banks to hold specific levels of cash reserves. However, it was the passage of the Futures Modernization Act in 2000 that completed the financialization of the US economy, by repealing all bans against single stock futures, and by prohibiting federal regulation of over-the-counter derivatives including the infamous mortgage-backed securities.
>
> (p. 19)

The economic shocks of the 2008 global financial crisis did the most health harm to those least responsible for the reckless financial gambling that created the crisis in the first place. As Mohindra and colleagues (2011) point out:

> although the global financial crisis began in the developed world, developing countries are the main victims ... In effect, poorer groups in poor countries (notably but not exclusively women) are bearing the brunt of unregulated financial speculation carried out by investment bankers in high income countries (notably but not exclusively men), whose 'rescue' by their governments has created a massive moral hazard[8] and public debt.
>
> (p. 282)

The moral hazard and public debt spawned by the financial crisis are references to how governments in HICs with sovereign currency (i.e. the ability to finance their debts without international borrowing) briefly abandoned neoliberal orthodoxy and used their central banks to 'print' (digitally create) trillions in new money to restart their economies. This 'quantitative easing' in the money supply temporarily saved capitalism from its own predations, but, in an unregulated global financial system, it also allowed new arbitrage fuel to fan new asset bubbles (De Vogli and Osuwu 2014), de facto rewarding the very ones responsible for the collapse. This brief (less than two-year) period of Keynesian counter-cyclical government spending was quickly followed by austerity, neoliberalism's third policy incarnation, a slightly less demanding form of earlier structural adjustment focusing primarily on reducing government debt, much of it newly created by the 2008 bailout.

Neoliberal governmentality

Before turning to austerity, another arm of critical public health scholarship on neoliberalism, and one popular with contributors to the *Journal of Critical Public Health* and its predecessors, directed its attention to neoliberalism's function as a disciplining governmentality (see also Chapter 5 of this volume). Ayo (2012), amongst others, describes how neoliberal governmentality had infiltrated health promotion practice. Drawing on the late French philosopher Michel Foucault's theorizing of "the ways in which humans come to engage in self-constituting practices", she writes that:

> ... governmentality was seen as a method of social control and political rule ... and key to this concept...within the context of contemporary neoliberalism is that such social control is neither deemed as being overtly coercive nor forceful, but rather as operating on autonomous individuals wilfully regulating themselves in the best interest of the state.
>
> (p. 100)

Neoliberalism in this sense is an exercise in hegemonic power, in which people so internalize its rationality that they act without direct coercion in ways that cohere with its basic tenets. As Ayo continues, this is consequent to how "neoliberalism as a system of thoughts and beliefs about the effective rule of state, society, and the market" had become "pervasive in that the corresponding discourses directly shape the ways in which society is governed and expected to conduct itself, right from the privacy of one's own home to the administration of public institutions and across all demographics" (p. 100).

The rise of 'healthism' in advanced economies, concomitant with the growth of a profitable health industry promoting products and services aimed at self-regulating the body, is seen as one example of such governmentality. So, too, is much health promotion practice with its emphasis on ill health as arising from poor individual choices, the 'lifestyle' focus that continues to 'drift' back into practice as earlier chapters described. Astute readers, however, may notice a slight contradiction in this alignment. On the one hand, individuals and their unhealthy behaviours become a focus of governmentality efforts to promote health and reduce the burden of chronic diseases, but at the same time "personal choice, and the freedom to choose" is regarded as "the very foundation of neoliberalism", a juxtaposition that conflates the idea of sovereign individual choice with the individuation of responsibility.

This contradiction resolves when the only rational choice for individuals to achieve their welfare-maximizing sovereignty is presumed to be investing in their own health and education, that is, enhancing their 'human capital' to assure their economic self-sufficiency. As Reubi (2016) points out, this is precisely what one school of neoliberal economics does, by embedding rational choice theory and microeconomics within the market fundamentalism of neoliberal macroeconomics. The role of the state in this regard is no longer one of promoting an ideology of 'healthism' or in disciplining those insisting on making the wrong choice; rather, it calls for public policy levers to direct personal choices towards health and human capital as the idealized rational choice. Thus, one finds neoliberal economists macroeconomically opposing government interventions while at the same time, and somewhat surprisingly, supporting government 'sin taxes' on unhealthy commodities (tobacco, alcohol, sugar) to decrease consumption. The resolving argument rests, in part, on acknowledging how (yet to be corrected) market failures lead to the costs of such consumption being borne by the state (anathema to neoliberal purists) rather than by individuals. This neoliberally ordained 'choice editing' of health behaviour may appear similar to health promotion's older invocation to use policy to 'make healthy choices the easy choices', but the rationality is different. Health is no longer the goal but simply an incidental pathway to the creation of (neoliberally) welfare-maximizing "entrepreneurs of themselves" (p. 483).

As Schrecker (2016a) argues, there is no contradiction between stating that there is an unhealthy 'neoliberal diet' while also claiming that neoliberal governmentality demands only healthy diets, whether or not prompted by sin taxes. Both describe facets of neoliberalization as a coherent programme. Flexibilizing labour markets and reducing welfare entitlements render healthy diets unaffordable for many, while deregulating global food industries allowing diffusion of cheap 'pseudo'-foods is consistent with neoliberalism's macroeconomic nostrums. Holding people personally accountable for sustaining a healthy diet is consistent with its microeconomic individuation of responsibility. Nonetheless, on a cautionary note, Schrecker concludes that:

> The postmodern turn in the academy … is conducive to scepticism about grand historical narratives, but that scepticism can be overdone if nuance and specificity are not accompanied by attention to macro-scale issues of context and power relations.
>
> (p. 479)

The globalization of austerity

That caution takes on more significance when considering neoliberalism's third macroeconomic iteration: austerity, which refers to governments' fiscal 'belt-tightening' to reduce public debt to avoid 'crowding out' (competing with) the private sector for access to capital. For many living in lower-middle-income countries (LMICs) and familiar with SAPs, the rapid shift from government bailout spending to fiscal retrenchment was nothing new; they had been living with some degree of austerity for decades. It was the extent of willing adoption of austerity by many HICs (or in the case of some EU member states, as a condition of bailouts by the 'troika' of the European Commission, European Central Bank, and IMF) that was novel. Although in some ways a fitting global response to a crisis of inherent global scale, what the near worldwide embrace of austerity revealed, more critically, was the tenacity with which neoliberal ideas survived despite their lack of empirical credibility. As Labonté (2012) points out:

> The stunning failure of the 2007 crisis[9] to 'starve the beast' of neoliberalism (whose tax cuts for wealthy individuals and corporations were meant to 'starve the beast' of government social spending) reveals the depth of public/private isomorphism. Neoliberalism was never about eliminating the state, it was about occupying it … The austerity agenda is merely one of the means.
>
> (p. 259)

Austerity is one of the pathways by which the 2008 financial crisis trickles down to cause poorer health outcomes. Drawing on earlier frameworks tracking globalization's many-layered policy impacts, one paper published in *Critical Public Health* in the post-crisis period modelled the 'health equity-relevant pathways' from crisis to differential health outcomes. Unlike systems or complexity frameworks with their two-tailed and positive/negative rankings of relationships, Ruckert and Labonté (2012) deliberately chose a one-tailed hierarchic model to elaborate on the extant evidence supporting the different components in the model and the direction of their effects (Figure 6.1). The two 'branches' of the pathways (direct and indirect influence) fit nicely with the two principal facets of neoliberalism just discussed: as macroeconomic policy and as microeconomic rationality. The article's 2012 conclusion "that the most challenging years are still ahead" was borne out by the post-2008 austerity-induced subsequent 'Great Recession', one which had barely receded before COVID-19 became the next disruptive crisis.

The immediate and acute negative health impacts of the 2008 financial crisis resemble those of earlier SAPs and include excess suicide mortality, a shift to less healthy eating and to more stress-coping unhealthy behaviours (smoking, binge drinking), and poorer healthcare access (Ruckert and Labonté 2014; Nour et al. 2017; Ruckert and Labonté 2017). But there is a different story to be told about the subsequent recession, which was not singularly damaging to health. The post-crisis recession did lead to unemployment, increased suicides, poorer nutrition, and generally poorer health for some, but De Vogli and Owusu (2014) also found that "with the exception of suicide rates, several studies have reported an overall reduction in mortality during times of economic recession", noting that:

> Although recessions are likely to be detrimental for individuals who lose their jobs, houses, and businesses, and for poor households that experience severe reductions in consumption levels, they are not necessarily unhealthy for the general population …
>
> (p. 22)

The caveat, of course, is that "favourable health outcomes in times of crises are more likely to be experienced by nations with stronger social protections" (p. 22) primarily those wealthier nations with the fiscal capacity to 'quantitatively ease' new money into creation to support *inter alia* income transfers, unemployment benefits, employment creation programmes, generous welfare rates, and public subsidies of healthy food and affordable housing. But, as de Vogli and Owusu point out, most of the $11.9 trillion in public funds was used to bail out the culprit banks

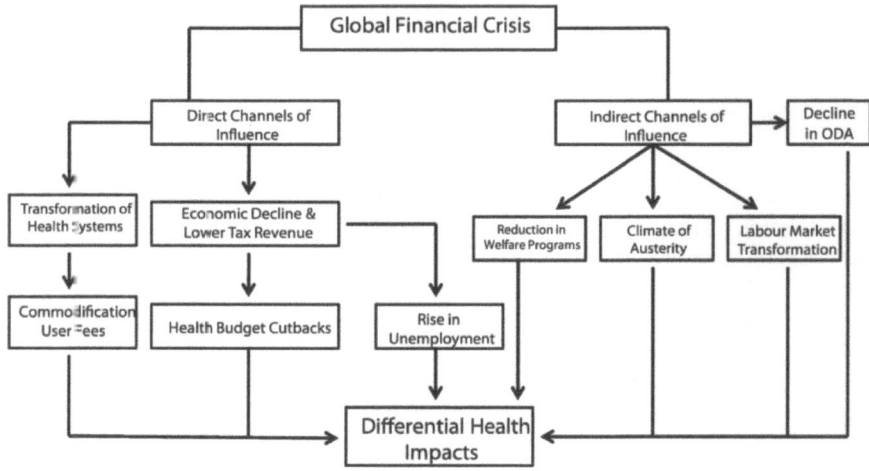

Figure 5.1 Pathways linking global financial crises to health outcomes.

(others place it as high as $14 trillion [Bank of England 2009]), leaving very little to support individuals left bearing the costs.

Unsurprisingly, the austerity measures immediately following the post-2008 crisis bailouts saw aggregate declines in health, education, and social spending in most countries (Ruckert and Labonté 2017). Moreover, echoing the indirect channels in Figure 6.1, transfers between rich and poor countries in the form of official development assistance (ODA) declined or stagnated. Subsequent declines in health and social spending in many sub-Saharan African (SSA) countries saw services demand transfer from cash-strapped government programmes to community-based organizations (CBOs). Akintola and colleagues (2015), in a qualitative study of health and social service CBOs in South Africa, found that most of these organizations also suffered a drop in donor funding, both international and domestic. This replicated the global financial crisis at very local levels, in many instances leading to staff retrenchments, attrition of volunteers, closure of some CBOs, reduced services, and a net decline in people's access to essential health and social care.

The IMF, chastened by the dismal growth returns of its earlier SAPs, argued that its post-2008 emergency funds to LICs came with fewer conditionalities. This is true, although left unsaid is the already very high levels of privatization or liberalization by that time and the question of how much more was even possible. In an internal assessment of its 2010 to 2017 loans, the IMF found that fiscal consolidation (spending cuts) was required in only half of the countries covered by one of its programmes. The assessment further noted that even when spending cuts were required, the loans stipulated protection of priority social protection budgets ('spending floors'). Stubbs and Kentikelenis (2018), in their independent review of the IMF assessment, challenged these findings as "methodologically flawed, unduly optimistic, and potentially misleading" (p. 133). Although their reassessment affirmed that there was no statistically significant impact on education spending in countries participating in an IMF programme over this time period, there was an association between IMF programme participation and decreased health spending. Spending floor requirements are non-binding, whereas requirements for fiscal contraction are binding. Failure to meet the binding requirements could imperil renewal of IMF financial assistance, creating a context in which " … macroeconomic targets set by the IMF crowd out health concerns" (p. 137).

Schrecker (2016b), in reviewing the UK's response to the financial crisis, emphasized that its austerity measures should be seen as "(a) selective, given continued budgeting of billions of pounds for questionably necessary transport and defence capital projects, and (b) not the only option in fiscal policy terms" (p. 8). He argues the importance of "interrogating scarcity" to oppose the critics of government social spending who claim it is unaffordable, citing a compelling example where:

> a bill aimed at improving food security in India was described by critics as 'financially irresponsible' when its officially estimated annual cost was approximately

half the revenue foregone each year by exempting imports of diamonds and gold from customs duties.

(p. 8)

Rather than austerity being seen as a necessity brought on by profligate public spending, it is best considered a political (ideological) choice that advances the longer-term neoliberal goal to "shrink the state, free up the market, and set ... political economy on a new course" (Schrecker 2016b, p. 8; Taylor-Gooby 2012).

Global austerity was in slight retreat until COVID-19 precipitated what is regarded as the greatest public health crisis since the 1918–1920 influenza pandemic. Many governments, as they did in the immediate aftermath of the 2008 financial crisis, responded with new rounds of 'quantitative easing', with central banks purchasing large amounts in government-issued bonds. Unlike 2008, however, and in response to public health mandated lockdowns to control disease spread prior to vaccine discovery, much of this new money went into income transfers and other subsidy programmes directed at individual workers and companies to keep domestic economies afloat, rather than singularly protecting banks.[10] In some instances, the supports to individuals were sufficiently generous that aggregate poverty rates and economic inequality declined during the lockdowns (as occurred in Canada and in the USA), even though poverty rates worsened globally. This generosity once more remained exclusive to HICs with their sovereign currencies and central banks. LMICs without such fiscal flexibilities had to borrow from international markets to offer support to their citizens, especially during the harsher early days of the pandemic (Labonté 2022).

This pandemic generosity was also time limited. As lockdown measures and other public health restrictions eventually eased, countries' 'quantitative easing' began shifting to 'quantitative tightening' as governments moved to reduce the amount of public debt being held by their central banks. Repeating the 2008 response, governments reimposed new rounds of austerity that, by late 2022, were estimated to affect 85% of the world's population, largely in developing countries. The depth of expenditure contraction in some countries is almost twice as great as it was following the 2008 crisis (Ortiz and Cummins 2021) and is projected to persist beyond 2025.

Free (unfair) trade

Trade is as old as human settlements and has been one of globalization's defining elements. Trade can generate positive or negative health impacts depending on who receives most of the trade-related benefits, such as income, resources, goods, and services, or is exposed to the bulk of its harms, including pollution, unemployment or poor working conditions, and damaging or dangerous goods. As Labonté (2019) wrote on this "ambivalent or dialectical relationship between trade and health":

There is nothing intrinsically unhealthy about international trade. Whether trade or foreign investment leads to health-enhancing or health-damaging outcomes related to social, economic, or regulatory changes depends very much on the specific and binding rules of particular agreements. Food trade can increase the availability, and even the affordability, of healthy foods but it can also flood markets with obesogenic (and more readily affordable) food products. Health services trade could improve the quality of care in many countries, but it could also increase privatization in such services and crowd out access for low-income populations. Intellectual property rights can incentivize new drug discoveries but price essential medicines beyond the affordability means of the poor or their governments. At an aggregate level, global trade can increase economic growth with potential trickle-down income growth and related health benefits, but not all countries will benefit equitably (if at all) and benefits within countries may be skewed in favour of some populations, but not others. To the extent that trade-related economic growth increases negative environmental externalities (such as climate change and resource depletion), it contributes indirectly to what are now increasingly central public health concerns. Trade rules could be used to further compliance with international environmental law, and to reduce barriers to the diffusion of 'green technologies'; but they can also be used (and have been) to challenge countries' subsidies or supports for the production and export of such technologies.

(p. 2/12)

Although trade as a critical public health issue received increased attention following the 1995 creation of the World Trade Organization (WTO) and the post-2000 surge in international investment agreements, there were relatively few studies explicitly focusing on trade and trade treaties in the journal *Critical Public Health*. Trade liberalization received passing comment in the first edition of this volume, with Labonté and Torgerson (2008) describing it as a "subset of macroeconomic policy" with the aim to "facilitate the reorganisation of production or commodity chains across national borders in order to maximise profitability" (p. 169). For public health advocates and civil society organizations, 'free' trade was increasingly regarded as 'unfair' trade, one in which trade treaties and their rules disproportionately benefited already developed countries and their corporate sector.

Since the twenty-teens, and the rise in bilateral or regional trade treaties bypassing stalled negotiations at the multilateral World Trade Organization (WTO), public health researchers have begun to turn their attention to the content of specific trade agreements. This immersion in trade's legal texts equipped public health advocates with the ability to infer future health benefits and losses, and equitable distribution therein, and to engage more effectively with the trade and finance sectors of governments that negotiate what are essentially commercial treaties. A primary focus of these recent trade studies was the Trans-Pacific Partnership Agreement (TPPA) (subsequently known as the Comprehensive and Progressive Trans-Pacific Partnership (CPTPP)) which, despite the withdrawal of the USA from negotiations in 2017, remains the largest free trade agreement outside the multilateral WTO. It is moot, however, whether the WTO will survive the unilateral trade/tariff practices of the second Trump administration, as described in the Conclusion chapter.

The paper by Ruckert et al. (2017) describes a health impact assessment (HIA) of what was then still referred to as the TPPA. The HIA relied on leaked texts

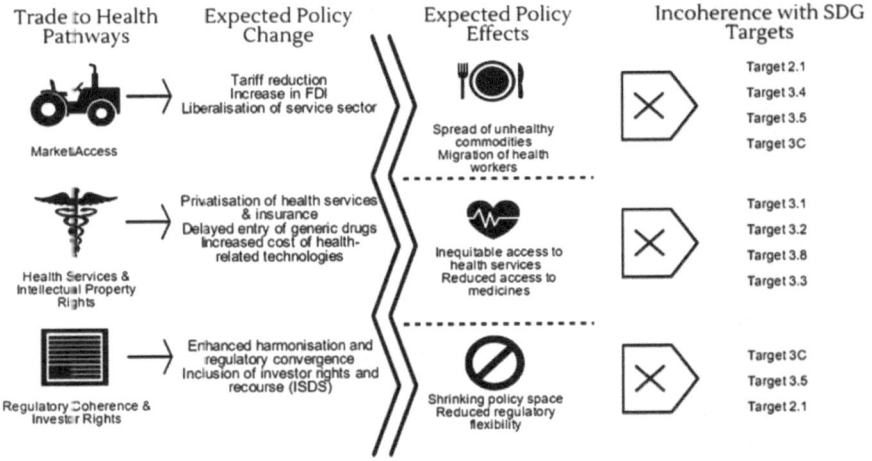

Figure 5.2 Conceptual framework for policy coherence analysis.

Source: Reprinted from Ruckert et al. 2017.

(trade negotiations are secretive), government statements, and already ratified treaties that indicated likely outcomes of the new agreement. Following accepted methods for HIAs, including screening, scoping, appraisal, and recommendations, the study began with a realist review of what was known about health effects of existing trade rules with an assumption that they would likely be strengthened in the TPPA. The specific intent of the HIA was to examine the extent to which TPPA provisions were likely to cohere with the 2015 Sustainable Development Goals (SDGs), which had been agreed upon by almost all the world's nations, along three specific pathways: unhealthy commodities, access to medicine, and regulatory flexibility (Figure 6.2). This last pathway reflected a growing concern amongst trade and health researchers and activists with the expansion of trade rules well beyond tariffs and subsidies, with rules that could dissuade governments from introducing health, environmental, or social policies that might, even inadvertently, dampen international trade or investment flows. Ruckert et al. found "that there is clear evidence that current trade and investment policy comes into tension, and in some cases directly conflict, with the SDGs" noting that:

> Although it is unlikely that all incoherences between policies in competing sectors can be eliminated, the managed reduction of potential policy incoherences will be essential to the global effort to achieve the SDGs.
>
> (p. 94)

Moreover, the authors argued that "achieving more health-sensitive trade policy requires increased recognition of corporate influence in trade negotiations and more salient efforts by health activists to counterbalance such influence" (p. 94).

One of the ways to counterbalance corporate influence is to gain a better understanding of how corporations frame trade policy in their interventions with government trade officials. Two TPPA-related health studies did that. The first, indicative of public health's long-standing concern with access to affordable medicines consequent to protectionist intellectual property rights (IPRs) in purportedly 'free' trade agreements, was a study of how the pharmaceutical industry used language and ideas to influence TPPA negotiations (Neuwelt et al. 2016). The research combined critical discourse, thematic, and policy analysis of publicly available texts produced by industry associations in the USA, which was, at that time, still part of TPPA negotiations, and New Zealand. Answering Bacchi's (1999) basic policy analysis question, 'What is the problem represented to be?' The researchers found that the industry personified itself as "the victim of unfair treatment, the protector of the public good, and economic saviour", all of which could and should be fixed via the TPPA. Industry submissions to trade officials argued that generic competition was inequitable and likely dangerous (the 'faking it' arguments by Erikson (2019), discussed earlier in this chapter) and that strong intellectual property protection increased the supply of life-saving drugs (a claim for which there is little actual evidence). In the case of the USA, strong IPRs for industry were seen as being in the nation's economic self-interest, "a finding that might explain why the industry has had privileged access to inside knowledge about the TPPA negotiations" (Neuwelt et al. 2016, p. 168).

A second study applied the same Bacchi framework to an analysis of food industry policy framing in four TPPA countries, Australia, New Zealand, Canada, and the USA (Friel et al. 2016). Five 'problem' themes were mobilized by food corporations, overlapping considerably with those of the pharmaceutical industry study. The TPPA, the food industry argued, would, first, bring economic and social benefits to member countries; second, improve WTO trade rules; third, increase market access, including for their exports, including processed foods; fourth, harmonize regulations amongst trading partners to increase trade flows; and fifth, ensure protection of foreign investment. Each of these industry claims is contentious. Although economic benefits are often claimed in political support of almost every new trade treaty, evidence shows that while some domestic sectors will gain, others will lose, and the net economic benefit is often negligible. This was later found to be the case with the TPPA (Labonté et al. 2016), as well as with the more recent USA/Mexico/Canada Agreement (USMCA) (Labonté et al. 2019).

Arguments by trade proponents to improve WTO rules speak to how powerful countries and their commercial interests are using bilateral and regional trade agreements strategically to wedge new measures benefiting transnational capital into the stalled multilateral system. Opening new markets for exported processed foods is of considerable public health concern: research has already demonstrated that trade agreements increase the market presence of unhealthy commodities, notably sugar-sweetened beverages (soda drinks) (Schram et al. 2015) and ultra-processed (high shelf-life) 'foods' (Stuckler et al. 2012). Foreign investment protection, ostensibly to prevent expropriation of investors' assets, has become a contentious and undemocratic system used by corporate and financial actors to prevent or 'chill' new government health and environment protection measures that could negatively affect the future value (profits) of their investments (Gleeson and Labonté 2020). Friel et al.'s (2016) conclusion emphasizes that "if coherence between trade and health policy goals is to be strengthened, the public health community will need to engage with industry arguments and build an effective counter-argument that gives prominence to health and nutritional concerns" (p. 528).

A third paper draws together key points from the studies described above, with a focus on all TPPA submissions made to the Australian government. Townsend et al. (2020) identified three distinct trade frames: a dominant neoliberal market frame, and two counter-frames, public interest and state sovereignty. The analysis focused on how differing frames relate to policies that improve social determinants of health, in much the same way that Ruckert et al. (2017) related their findings to the SDGs. The market frame, which was invoked almost entirely by industry actors, "was particularly constraining for arguments to address the social determinants of health" (p. 119), whereas the public interest frame favoured by civil society organizations argued for the importance of placing "public social and health interests above market interests" (p. 120). The final frame, state sovereignty, "challenges the dominant market frame in which the state's role is primarily defined as facilitating economic growth, to one which emphasizes the need to protect the right of states to regulate in the public interest" (p. 121). None of the industry submissions, which far outnumbered the rest, made any reference to public interest or state sovereignty concerns. Repeating earlier arguments concerning neoliberal hegemony, Townsend et al. noted (2020):

The assumptions underpinning free market trade and unfettered liberalisation are so pervasive amongst trade policy discussions that, despite evidence of counter-frames by civil society and health groups, the market/economic remit continues to dominate trade and investment discussions.

(p. 123)

Yet, the study also concludes that opportunities for critical public health exist, notably, opportunities for:

… more explicit engagement and critique of the assumptions underpinning the market frame ... [engaging] with heterodox economic studies that document the failures of 'trickle down' economics to generate wellbeing …

(p. 123)

This is happening. Many contributors to the *Journal of Critical Public Health* and its earlier iterations are engaging with heterodox economists, but also with trade negotiators, by learning their language in order to better contextualize health equity issues within trade and investment treaties. They continue undertaking studies that assess the impacts of trade flows and treaty rules on population health outcomes (e.g. Barlow et al. 2017; Barlow et al. 2018). They are working alongside trade and eco-justice networks, supporting the claims of rural and Indigenous communities that are mobilizing against the toxic extractive capitalism abetted by trade and investment treaties (Labonté and Bodini 2022). *Critical Public Health* never became the major outlet for many of these studies, given the number of journals where globalization, trade, and health are more clearly defined niche areas.[11] But, despite claims that the COVID-19 pandemic, alongside geopolitical tensions (the US/China competition for the role of global hegemon and Russia's invasion of Ukraine), is ending the neoliberal trade era, and notwithstanding evidence of US-led re-emergent protectionism (see also the Conclusion chapter of this volume), during the early 2020s global trade flows continued to rise (UNCTAD 2022), as did the number of new bilateral or regional trade treaties. Trade may be reconfiguring along 'near-shoring' or 'friend-shoring' lines, which could provoke trade wars (Labonté et al. 2022) and with Trump's second presidency, as the Conclusion chapter notes, it already has; but this simply signals a need for more, and more critical, public health attention to the trade/health relationship now than in the recent past.

Commercial/corporate determinants of health

The role of trade and investment treaties in incentivizing the global diffusion of unhealthy commodities represents one aspect of what are now often called the 'commercial' (or more recently, the 'corporate') determinants of health. These determinants thread back through trade and economic globalization, as two studies published in *Critical Public Health* document. In one study. De Vogli and colleagues (2011) examined the correlation between the number of one fast-food outlet (Subway) per 100,000 population and male/female body mass index (BMI)/obesity rates in 26 of 34 advanced economies. Diffusion of that fast-food outlet, partly attributed to trade and investment liberalization policies, was associated with increased rates of overweight and obesity in the long term and high intake of sugars, fats, salt, and other 'unhealthy' components of processed/ultra-processed foods in the short term. While study design (ecological, cross-sectional) precludes inference of causality, the results are consistent with other aggregate-level studies that show associations between fast-food restaurants and obesity prevalence, yet in this case the findings were, importantly, situated within the commercial or corporate context of economic globalization.

A second study (De Vogli et al. 2014) used time-series and longitudinal cross-national analysis of 127 countries (1980–2008) to explore whether BMI is affected by economic globalization and inequality. The study used the KOF index of economic globalization, which relies upon a number of variables related to trade and investment flows.[12] The study found a statistically significant relationship between increases in economic globalization and body-mass index (BMI) after adjusting for GDP per capita, urbanization, population size, and within-country inequality. The researchers suggest that economic inequality may play a role but "the exact mechanisms … remain to be clarified" (p. 18) with some evidence that liberalized investment allowing for the worldwide proliferation of transnational food corporations may be a more important factor in the diffusion of highly processed food, soft drinks, and fast food than trade in unhealthy commodities per se.[13]

Other Big Food studies focus less on trade or investment and more on corporate marketing practices to explain the global increase in obesity and associated diseases (Williams and Nestle 2015). There is a conventional belief that the 'nutrition transition' occurring in most LMICs is an inevitable outcome of economic development and the increased global availability of sugars, meats, fats, and oil. Westernized diets of processed and fast foods are aggressively marketed and consumed, viewed as symbols of success and social status. Basu (2015) found mixed evidence for this narrative, with some countries following the convention, others following it but with some nuance (little increase in meats but a rise in local edible oils also harmful to cardiovascular health and, with palm oil, to ecosystems), and a few others bucking most of these trends altogether. Data limitations preclude any final assessment as to why there is such variability in Big Food outcomes, but Basu's study contends that government policy choices likely play an important role. This inference has reinforcement in a mixed-methods analysis of Big Food's presence in Kenya (O'Neill 2015), a country that, like others in the region, has experienced a large influx of transnational and localized fast-food outlets alongside a growth in supermarkets with abundant processed (and inexpensive) food items. As the authors reflect:

> Based on this picture, it would seem plausible to expect that major dietary changes are underway in Kenya ... Yet the dietary profiles for Kenya do not reflect such an obvious change.
>
> (p. 267)

While edible oil consumption may be problematic for healthy dietary reasons, a related study (Downs et al. 2022) found that per capita meat and sugar consumption had changed little in Kenya since the early 1960s. This finding was attributed, in part, to government policies that regulated oil, sugar, and other food staple supplies to support national food self-sufficiency. The study forewarned that a shift to less healthy food consumption patterns remains, "particularly as domestic protections expire, or if factory farming gains a foothold" (p. 273).[14]

A different approach to Big Food examined industry efforts to influence scientific evidence and opinion in the health/nutrition nexus (Sacks et al. 2018). The contributors describe how industry officials adopt well-known tactics deployed for decades by the tobacco industry: they emphasize individual choice (the neoliberal default), infiltrate policymaking, lobby and bankroll politicians, skirt regulation by queuing corporate social responsibility, commission counter-research, and use 'social aspect' or 'front' organizations to advance these strategies (Oreskes 2010). The study, published in *Critical Public Health*, is only one of many to have investigated food industry influence on media, regulators, and policymakers, undertaken collaboratively with the 'US Right to Know' NGO. As of 2022, at least 16 papers had been published in peer-reviewed journals, relying primarily on content analyses of publicly released email exchanges between industry officials, regulators, and industry-financed and nominally independent organizations (U.S. Right to Know 2023). These studies draw on multiple emails, internal memos, and published reports, with links to the public data files used in the analyses to demonstrate rigour and transparency.[15]

With respect to alcohol or 'Big Booze', another of the triad of unhealthy commodities, Herrick (2016) finds that public health criticisms of alcohol as an 'industrial epidemic' are still modest compared to those concerning tobacco and food and urges new approaches to alcohol/health research to inform regulatory advocacy. She is specifically concerned with a perceived ideological schism within the health research community itself, between those taking a tobacco-like hard line against alcohol (no contact at all with industry) and others emphasizing a more moderate stance involving research collaboration, funding, and co-working within policy development; in other words, the very practices interrogated and critiqued by the Big Food studies described above. Cautioning against too firm a boundary between research and industry, Herrick contends that "it is hard to imagine any reasoned 'science' emerging from a politics in which industry contact with research(ers) is almost always cast as 'contentious' or ... 'moral jeopardy'" but that "without contact there can be little basis for knowledge generation or evidence on which to base advocacy" (Herrick 2016, p. 17). Unlike tobacco, there is no framework convention (a reference to the WHO Framework Convention on Tobacco Control) to delineate conflict-of-interest boundaries, and, unlike food, there are no legal suits creating archives of corporate documents rich for public health scrutiny. Although not all critical health researchers might agree with Herrick's argument, most would likely concur with her conclusion that bad public health policy decisions regarding 'industrial epidemics' are not simply the result of industry interference but rather reflect a constellation of ideological, professional, and epistemological factors that we discuss throughout this volume.

The third of our industrial epidemics – tobacco – is the one with the longest history of public health critique. Scores of tobacco-related articles have appeared in *Critical Public Health*, and tobacco control has its own specialized journal (BMJ *Tobacco Control*). Increasingly, the focus on tobacco has shifted from health-specific (or at least health-reductive) studies, or those evaluating health behaviour interventions, to greater attention on industry practices, with a subset drawing on political economy theory. In an article focusing on Zambia, one of SSA's tobacco-growing countries, Ruckert et al. (2023) argue that applying a political economy lens "offers an entry point into analysing the complex relationship between the political and economic actors involved in tobacco production and control" (p. 31). Their paper, a mixed-methods analysis of interviews and government and tobacco industry reports, challenges the Big Tobacco discourse of the importance of tobacco farming to poverty reduction and economic development in LMICs, concluding that:

> ... the narrative of tobacco's benefit to the micro- and macro-economy is perpetuated by entrenched interests and taken up by government sectors working with misinformation and under a narrow framing [in] a context with limited alternatives. This context is structured by a longstanding history of tobacco growing and an institutionalization of tobacco in government, as well

as the broader structural conditions of the global economy, namely the push for export-oriented cash crops, the dwindling of government support for and privatization of supply chains, and the concentration of power among transnational corporations.

(p. 31)

Their paper is part of a decade-long set of studies in five SSA countries that aim to deconstruct the claim made by industry and often parroted by governments (or some sectors therein) that tobacco is essential to rural farming livelihoods. Detailed multi-wave surveys of rural tobacco and non-tobacco farming households in these countries, combined with focus group data, find that most tobacco-growing households are bound within contracts that often leave them in debt at the end of a growing season, thereby replicating an impoverishing dependency cycle. Superficially, the payments tobacco farmers receive at the end of a growing season, under the guaranteed payments contract, do supply the household with some cash in hand. But when monetizing all inputs into tobacco production, including the value of unpaid household labour, most tobacco-growing households are found to earn very little or nothing at all. As one of the group's studies on Malawi, the most tobacco-dependent country amongst the five, noted (Makola 2017):

> In 2011 [the year the studies began], two of the largest European tobacco firms, British American Tobacco (BAT) and Imperial Tobacco, had profit margins of 34% and 39% respectively. By implication, the high profit margins of the tobacco transnationals are in part a function of the impoverishing unpaid labour of tobacco farmers' households.

(pp. 38–39)

Microeconomic analyses and political economy critiques of the tobacco livelihood argument have resonated amongst government policymakers. Drawing attention to who profits, and who pays for those profits, across a spectrum of corporate commodities is also gaining critical public health attention. Wood and colleagues (2023), in a macroeconomic analysis, examine trends in corporate wealth and income distribution in four unhealthy commodity industries (UCIs): fossil fuels (for which more critical public health research is needed), tobacco, alcohol, and ultra-processed foods. Amongst their key findings:

1 Effective corporate tax rates for the UCIs have fallen by half or more since the post-1980 neoliberal era;
2 The adjusted value of UCI dividend payments and share repurchases (which increase the value of shares that comprise part of corporate executive pay packages) tripled from the 1960s to the late 2000s;
3 Most of those benefiting from this surge in income reside in HICs.

The authors describe these outcomes as a 'double burden of maldistribution', in which "[UCIs'] externalised social and ecological harms disproportionately affect disadvantaged population groups and governments in low- and middle-income countries; whilst, simultaneously, they are increasingly transferring wealth and income to a group over-represented by a small and privileged elite" (Wood et al. 2023, p. 135).

Conclusion: the question of governance

One idea that threads throughout the themes in this chapter is that, as the Commission on Social Determinants of Health (2008) stated, it is "the toxic combination of poor social policies, unfair economics, and bad politics [that] is responsible for much of health inequity" (p. 35). The political and economic decisions made by powerful elite groups and actors give too little heed to the health (and health equity) consequences of their choices. Are our current systems of governance (the rules, norms, laws, and institutions that oversee organized societies) capable of ensuring a fair and healthy future?

Notes

1 Until the 1970s, it was common to divide the world into categories based on Western concepts of 'development' based on industrialization, income, and life expectancy: developed (high levels), developing countries (low levels), and least developed (very low levels). These designations, while still frequently used, were criticized for their implicit assumptions of what constituted development (primarily extractive industrial growth) and for the extent of national variance within each category. The World Bank (WB) in 1978 began to use income-based categories, dividing the world into four categories – high, upper middle, lower middle, and low – using an adjusted cost of an essential basket of goods (The World Bank 2019). While allowing for a more nuanced categorization, the WB system still relies on national-level comparisons and economic measures that give little insight into income distribution within countries or to the quality of people's lives (their 'lived experiences'). Depending on context, both categorical systems (developed/developing and income-grouping) are used in this chapter.

2 Although the global south/north dichotomy is still commonly used and captures the persisting large geographic inequalities in health resources, it should not obscure the rise in wealth inequities that are increasingly common in both hemispheres.

3 The International Health Regulations (IHRs) are international legal instruments binding on 196 countries, including the 194 WHO member states, and create rights and obligations with respect to control of epidemic and pandemic disease threats. In response to the COVID-19 pandemic, a process to review and revise the IHRs was initiated in 2022 and completed in 2024, although these have not yet been ratified by all member states. Apart from non-adopting countries, the 2024 amended IHRs will enter into force in September 2025. Non-adopting countries, including the USA, will still be bound by the 2005 IHRs.

4 We return to these financing issues in global health return in the next chapter, in a discussion of global governance in the wake of COVID-19 (IHR reform and a new pandemic accord).

5 The journal *Critical Public Health* is one of many that quickly published thoughtful commentaries summarizing the work of the Commission and assessing its historic importance, including the article by Baum (2008). See also Chapter 4 of this volume.

6 Elite and business interests also lobbied aggressively for a neoliberal shift, having watched their share of economic wealth decline under Keynesianism. As one political economist argued: "The hidden agenda of the Reagan/Thatcher revolution was to reverse this 'Great Compression' and allow income and wealth to be restored to their rightful owners at the top – combining market liberalization with an array of state measures which had the effect, intended and unintended, of intensifying redistribution upwards" (Wade 2009).

7 Hayek, an Australian economist whose later time at the University of Chicago influenced a generation of libertarian economist, like Milton Friedman, was motivated by a concern that some amalgam of (then rising) communism, socialism, and social democracy would lead to totalitarianism. Keynes, his economic rival, shared the same worry over totalitarianism but believed that the volatility of unfettered capitalism and unregulated markets was more likely to lead to this outcome.

8 In economics, a moral hazard is when public policy responses that 'bail out' market failures create an expectation that similar failures in the future will also be publicly rescued, usually by public debt-financed spending.

9 The global financial crisis is sometimes pegged as starting in 2007, when some banks or hedge funds began declaring bankruptcy, although most analysts consider 2008 to be more accurate in capturing the year when it became truly global in scale.

10 A US study, however, estimated that government COVID-19 support to American families and firms indirectly benefitted banks by between \$100 and \$300 billion by covering loan payments and preventing bank losses (Feldman and Schmidt 2021). One might assume indirect bank benefits in other countries enacting similar public financing support. Moreover, considerable support went to firms not necessarily needing it and not always passing on the public largesse to their employees. In the USA, only one-fifth of the government's 2020 COVID-19 bailouts went to individuals, with over half going to businesses, many of which did not need the cash (Whoriskey et al. 2020).

11 See, for example, the Trade and Health Collection here: www.biomedcentral.com/coll ections/trade-health

12 The KOF index (KOF refers to the economic research institute, *Konjunkturforschungsstelle)* measures the economic, social, and political dimensions of globalization. The economic sub-index focuses on trade- and investment-related measures and regulations (Dreher 2006).

13 Gleeson and Labonté (2020), in their review of different methodologies used to interrogate the trade/health relationship, note that 'big data' studies often yield inconsistent results, albeit generally finding negative health impacts. Discrepancies arise from limitations inherent to most such studies, even when trade agreements are the independent variable and aggregate health and/or nutrition outcomes are the dependent variables. Causality is rarely claimed, apart from rare instances of 'natural experiments' that allow for analysis of pre/post effects with matched country comparisons. Most trade/health review articles conclude by noting the "importance of complementary study designs, including more detailed and nuanced case studies of particular countries, comparative studies of particular globalisation and trade openness pathways, and theoretical, descriptive, and qualitative research" (p. 143).

14 This recent paper on food environments in informal settlements in Nairobi by Downs et al. 2022 suggests that the high cost of meats and commercially processed foods coupled with the availability of fruits and vegetables may be sustaining a reasonably diverse and healthy Kenyan food environment.

15 The study published in *Critical Public Health* (Sacks et al. 2018) reviewed a single email exchange to provide "a high-level perspective on the operations of the food

industry in relation to the debate around diet and nutrition" (p. 257). As journal editors, our preference would be to see more data-rich analyses to minimize the (almost invariable) pushback from industry that is directed against authors and journals that publish such critiques. It is also interesting to note that Sacks et al.'s public interest partnership between university researchers and civil society activists essentially mirrors industry's use of research and policy argumentation, albeit to challenge, rather than to promote, industry's private interests.

References

Akintola, O. *et al.* (2015) 'The global financial crisis: experiences of and implications for community-based organizations providing health and social services in South Africa', *Critical Public Health*, 26(3), pp. 307–321. Available at: https://doi.org/10.1080/09581 596.2015.1085959

Allman, D. (2019) 'Pseudo or perish: problematizing the "predatory" in global health publishing', *Critical Public Health*, 29(4), pp. 413–423. Available at: https://doi.org/ 10.1080/09581596.2019.1606417

Ayo, N. (2012) 'Understanding health promotion in a neoliberal climate and the making of health conscious citizens', *Critical Public Health*, 22(1), pp. 99–105. Available at: https:// doi.org/10.1080 /09581596.2010.520692

Bank of England (2009) *Financial Stability Report*. 25. Available at: www.bankofengland. co.uk /-/media/boe/files/financial-stability-report/2009/june-2009.pdf

Barlow, P., McKee, M. and Stuckler, D. (2018) 'The impact of U.S. free trade agreements on calorie availability and obesity: a natural experiment in Canada', *American Journal of Preventive Medicine*, 54(5), pp. 637–643. Available at: https://doi.org/10.1016/j.ame pre.2018.02.010

Barlow, P. *et al.* (2017) 'The health impact of trade and investment agreements: a quantitative systematic review and network co-citation analysis', *Globalization and Health*, 13(1), p. 13. Available at: https://doi.org/10.1186/s12992-017-0240-x

Basu, S. (2015) 'The transitional dynamics of caloric ecosystems: changes in the food supply around the world', *Critical Public Health*, 25(3), pp. 248–264. Available at: https://doi. org/10.1080/09581596.2014.931568

Bell, K. and Green, J. (2016). On the perils of invoking neoliberalism in public health critique. *Critical Public Health*, 26(3), pp. 239–243. Available at: https://doi.org/10.1080/ 09581596.2016.1144872

Commission on Social Determinants of Health (2008) 'Closing the gap in a generation: health equity through action on the social determinants of health' Geneva, Switzerland: WHO. Available at: /www.who.int/publications/i/item/WHO-IER-CSDH-08.1

De Vogli, R., Kouvonen, A. and Gimeno, D. (2011) '"Globesization": ecological evidence on the relationship between fast food outlets and obesity among 26 advanced economies', *Critical Public Health*, 21(4), pp. 395–402. Available at: https://doi.org/10.1080/09581 596.2011.619964

De Vogli, R. and Owusu, J.T. (2014) 'The causes and health effects of the Great Recession: from neoliberalism to "healthy de-growth"', *Critical Public Health*, 25(1), pp. 15–31. Available at: https://doi.org /10.1080/09581596.2014.957164.

De Vogli, R. *et al.* (2014) 'Economic globalization, inequality and body mass index: a cross-national analysis of 127 countries', *Critical Public Health*, 24(1), pp. 7–21. Available at: https://doi.org/10.1080 /09581596.2013.768331

Downs, S.M. *et al.* (2022) 'Food environments and their influence on food choices: a case study in informal settlements in Nairobi, Kenya', *Nutrients*, 14(13), p. 2571. Available at: https://doi.org/10.3390 /nu14132571

Dreher, A. (2006) 'Does globalization affect growth? Evidence from a new index of globalization', *Applied Economics*, 38(10), pp. 1091–1110. Available at: https://doi.org/10.1030/00036840500392078

Erikson, S. (2019) 'Faking global health', *Critical Public Health*, 29(4), pp. 508–516. Available at: https://doi.org/10.1080/09581596.2019.1601159

Feldmar, R. and Schmidt, J. (2021) 'Government fiscal support protected banks from huge losses during the COVID-19 crisis', *Federal Reserve Bank of Minneapolis*, 26 May. Available at: www.minneapolisfed.org/article/2021/government-fiscal-support-protec ted-banks-from-huge-losses-during-the-covid-19-crisis

Ferguson, J. (2010) The uses of neoliberalism. *Antipode*, 41(S1), 166–184.10.1111/anti.2010.41.issue-s1

Friel, S. *et al.* (2016) 'Shaping the discourse: What has the food industry been lobbying for in the Trans Pacific Partnership trade agreement and what are the implications for dietary health?', *Critical Public Health*, 26(5), pp. 518–529. Available at: https://doi.org/10.1030/09581596.2016.1139689

Gleeson, D. and Labonté, R. (2020) *Trade agreements and public health: a primer for health policy makers, researchers and advocates*. London: Palgrave.

Green, J. and Labonté, R. (eds) (2008) *Critical perspectives in public health*. London: Routledge.

Herrick, C. (2016) 'Alcohol, ideological schisms and a science of corporate behaviours on health', *Critical Public Health*, 26(1), pp. 14–23. Available at: https://doi.org/10.1080/09581596.2014.951313

Hodges, S. (2019). 'The case of the 'Spurious Drugs Kingpin': Shifting pills in Chennai, India', *Critical Public Health*, 29(4), 473–483.

Hodgson, C. (2020) 'World Bank ditches second round of pandemic bonds.' Available at: www.ft.com/content/949adc20-5303-494b-9cf1-4eb4c8b6aa6b (Accessed: 11 June 2025).

Jonas, C. (2019) 'Pandemic bonds: designed to fail in Ebola', *Nature*, 572(7769), pp. 285–285. Available at: https://doi.org/10.1038/d41586-019-02415-9

Kingori, P. and Gerrets, R. (2019) 'Why the pseudo matters to global health', *Critical Public Health*, 29(4), pp. 379–389. Available at: https://doi.org/10.1080/09581596.2019.1605155

Koplan, J.P. *et al.* (2009) 'Towards a common definition of global health', *The Lancet*, 373(9679), pp. 1993–1995. Available at: https://doi.org/10.1016/S0140-6736(09)60332-9

Labonté, R. (2008) 'Introduction to Part III. Colonising places: public health and globalisation', in J. Green and R. Labonté (eds.) *Critical Perspectives in Public Health*. London: Routledge, pp. 136–149.

Labonté, R. (2012) 'The austerity agenda: How did we get here and where do we go next?', *Critical Public Health*, 22(3), pp. 257–265. Available at: https://doi.org/10.1080/09581596.2012.687508

Labonté, R. (2019) 'Trade, investment and public health: compiling the evidence, assembling the arguments', *Globalization and Health*, 15(1), pp. 1, s12992-018-0425-y. Available at: https://doi.org/10.1186 /s12992-018-0425-y

Labonté, R. (2022) 'Ensuring global health equity in a post-pandemic economy', *International Journal of Health Policy and Management*, 11(8), pp. 1246–1250. Available at: https://doi.org/10.34172/ijhpm.2022.7212

Labonte, R. and Bodini, C. (2022) *In the shadow of the pandemic*. London [England]: Bloomsbury Academic Press (Global Health Watch, 6). Available at: https://doi.org/10.5040/9781350320840

Labonté, R., Martin, G. and Storeng, K.T. (2022) 'Editorial: whither globalization and health in an era of geopolitical uncertainty?', *Globalization and Health*, 18(1), pp. 87, s12992-022-00881–x. Available at: https://doi.org/10.1186/s12992-022-00881-x

Labonté, R. and Ruckert, A. (2019) *Health equity in a globalizing era: past challenges, future prospects*. First edition. Oxford New York: Oxford University Press.

Labonté, R., Schram, A. and Ruckert, A. (2016) 'The Trans-Pacific Partnership Agreement and health: few gains, some losses, many risks', *Globalization and Health*, 12(1), p. 25. Available at: https://doi.org/10.1186 /s12992-016-0166-8

Labonté, R and Schrecker, T. (2007). 'Globalization and the social determinants of health: Introduction and methodological background' (part 1 of 3) *Globalization and Health*, 3(5), 1–10.

Labonté, R. and Torgerson, R. (2008) 'Interrogating globalisation, health and development: towards a comprehensive framework for research, policy and political action", in J. Green and R. Labonté (eds.). *Critical Perspectives in Public Health*. London: Routledge, pp. 162–179.

Labonté, R. *et al.* (2019) 'USMCA (NAFTA 2.0): tightening the constraints on the right to regulate for public health', *Globalization and Health*, 15(1), p. 35. Available at: https://doi.org/10.1186/s12992-019-0476-8

Lambert, J. (2019) 'Bottle of lies' exposes the dark side of the generic-drug boom', *NPR*. Available at: www.npr.org/sections/health-shots/2019/05/12/722216512/bottle-of-lies-exposes-the-dark-side-of-the- generic-drug-boom (Accessed: 17 February 2023).

Lange, J. (2022) 'Removing author fees can help open access journals make research available to everyone', *The Conversation (online)*, 15 September. Available at: https://theconversation.com/removing-author-fees-can-help-open-access-journals-make-research-available-to-everyone-189675 (Accessed: 17 February 2023).

Larkin, M. (2008) 'Globalisation and health', in J. Green and R. Labonté (eds.) *Critical Perspectives in Public Health*. London: Routledge, pp. 151–161.

Light, D.W., Lexchin, J. and Darrow, J.J. (2013) 'Institutional corruption of pharmaceuticals and the myth of safe and effective drugs', *Journal of Law, Medicine & Ethics*, 41(3), pp. 590–600. Available at: https://doi.org/10.1111/jlme.12068

Makoka, D. *et al.* (2017) 'Costs, revenues and profits: an economic analysis of smallholder tobacco farmer livelihoods in Malawi', *Tobacco Control*, 26(6), pp. 634–640. Available at: https://doi.org/10.1136 /tobaccocontrol-2016-053022

Mohindra, K.S., Labonté, R. and Spitzer, D. (2011) 'The global financial crisis: whither women's health?', *Critical Public Health*, 21(3), pp. 273–287. Available at: https://doi.org/10.1080/09581596.2010.539593

Montenegro, C.R., Bernales, M. and Gonzalez-Aguero, M. (2020) 'Teaching global health from the south: challenges and proposals', *Critical Public Health*, 30(2), pp. 127–129. Available at: https://doi.org/10.1080 /09581596.2020.1730570

Neuwelt, P.M., Gleeson, D. and Mannering, B. (2016) 'Patently obvious: a public health analysis of pharmaceutical industry statements on the Trans-Pacific Partnership international trade agreement', *Critical Public Health*, 26(2), pp. 159–172. Available at: https://doi.org/10.1080/09581596.2015.1022510

Nour, S., Labonté, R. and Bancej, C. (2017) 'Impact of the 2008 global financial crisis on the health of Canadians: repeated cross-sectional analysis of the Canadian Community

Health Survey, 2007–2013', *Journal of Epidemiology and Community Health*, 71(4), pp. 336–343. Available at: https://doi.org/10.1136 /jech-2016-207661

O'Neill, K. (2015) 'Big Food without big diets? Food regimes and Kenyan diets', *Critical Public Health*, 25(3), pp. 265–279. Available at: https://doi.org/10.1080/09581 596.2015.1007922

Oreskes. N. and Conway, E.M. (2010) *Merchants of doubt: how a handful of scientists obscured the truth on issues from tobacco smoke to climate change.* Paperback edition, Nachdruck. New York London Oxford New Delhi Sydney: Bloomsbury.

Ortiz, I. and Cummins, M. (2021) *Global austerity alert looming budget cuts in 2021-25 and alternative pathways: working paper.* New York: Initiative for Policy Dialogue. Available at: https://policydialogue.org /files/publications/papers/Global-Austerity-Alert-Ortiz-Cummins-2021-final.pdf

Reubi, D. (2016) 'Of neoliberalism and global health: human capital, market failure and sin/social taxes', *Critical Public Health*, 26(5), pp. 481–486. Available at: https://doi.org/ 10.1080/09581596.2016.1196288

Ruckert, A. and Labonté, R. (2012) 'The global financial crisis and health equity: toward a conceptual framework', *Critical Public Health*, 22(3), pp. 267–279. Available at: https:// doi.org/10.1080 /09581596.2012.685053

Ruckert, A. and Labonté, R. (2014) 'The global financial crisis and health equity: early experiences from Canada', *Globalization and Health*, 10(1), p. 2. Available at: https://doi. org/10.1186/1744-8603-10-2

Ruckert, A. and Labonté, R. (2017) 'Health inequities in the age of austerity: the need for social protection policies', *Social Science & Medicine*, 187, pp. 306–311. Available at: https://doi.org/10.1016 /j.socscimed.2017.03.029

Ruckert, A. *et al.* (2017) 'Policy coherence, health and the sustainable development goals: a health impact assessment of the Trans-Pacific Partnership', *Critical Public Health*, 27(1), pp. 85–96. Available at: https://doi.org/10.1080/09581596.2016.1178379

Ruckert, A. *et al.* (2023) 'Exploring the political economy nexus of tobacco production and control: a case study from Zambia', *Critical Public Health*, 33(1), pp. 25–36. Available at: https://doi.org/10.1080 /09581596.2021.1981540

Rushton, S. and Williams, O.D. (2012) 'Frames, paradigms and power: global health policy-making under neoliberalism', *Global Society*, 26(2), pp. 147–167. Available at: https:// doi.org/10.1080 /13600826.2012.656266

Sacks, G. *et al.* (2018) 'How food companies influence evidence and opinion – straight from the horse's mouth', *Critical Public Health*, 28(2), pp. 253–256. Available at: https://doi. org/10.1080 /09581596.2017.1371844

Schram, A. *et al.* (2015) 'The role of trade and investment liberalization in the sugar-sweetened carbonated beverages market: a natural experiment contrasting Vietnam and the Philippines', *Globalization and Health*, 11(1), p. 41. Available at: https://doi.org/ 10.1186/s12992-015-0127-7

Schrecker, T. (2016a) '"Neoliberal epidemics" and public health: sometimes the world is less complicated than it appears', *Critical Public Health*, 26(5), pp. 477–480. Available at: https://doi.org/10.1080 /09581596.2016.1184229

Schrecker, T. (2016b) 'Globalization, austerity and health equity politics: taming the inequality machine, and why it matters', *Critical Public Health*, 26(1), pp. 4–13. Available at: https://doi.org/10.1080 /09581596.2014.973019

Stuckler, D. McKee, M. Ebrahim, S. and Basu, S. (2012) Manufacturing epidemics: The role of global producers in increased consumption of unhealthy commodities including

processed foods, alcohol, and tobacco. *PLoS Medicine*, 9(6), p. e1001235. https://doi.org/
10.1371/ journal. pmed.1001235

Structural Adjustment Participatory Review International Network (SAPRIN) (2002) *The
policy roots of economic crisis and poverty: A multi- country participatory assessment of
structural adjustment*. Washington, DC: SAPRIN. Available at: www.saprin.org/SAPR
IN_Findings.pdf

Stubbs, T. and Kentikelenis, A. (2018) 'Targeted social safeguards in the age of universal
social protection: the IMF and health systems of low-income countries', *Critical Public
Health*, 28(2), pp. 132–139. Available at: https://doi.org/10.1080/09581596.2017.1340589

Taylor-Gooby, P. (2012) 'Root and branch restructuring to achieve major cuts: the social
policy programme of the 2010 UK coalition government', *Social Policy & Administration*,
46(1), pp. 61–82. Available at: https://doi.org/10.1111/j.1467-9515.2011.00797.x

The World Bank (2019) 'Classifying countries by income', *World Bank (online)*, 9
September. Available at: https://datatopics.worldbank.org/world-development-indicators/
stories/the-classification-of-countries-by-income.html (Accessed: 17 February 2023).

Townsend, B. *et al.* (2020) 'How does policy framing enable or constrain inclusion of social
determinants of health and health equity on trade policy agendas?', *Critical Public Health*,
30(1), pp. 115–126. Available at: https://doi.org/10.1080/09581596.2018.1509059

UNCTAD (2022) *Global Trade Update*. Geneva: UNCTAD. Available at: https://unctad.
org/system/files /official-document/ditcinf2022d4_en.pdf

UNDESA (2006) *World Economic and Social Survey 2006 Diverging Growth and
Development*. United Nations. Available at: www.un.org/development/desa/dpad/publicat
ion/world-economic-and-social-survey-2006/

U.S. Right to Know (2023) 'Pursuing truth and transparency for public health (online)'.
Available at: https://usrtk.org/academic-work/ (Accessed: 17 February 2023).

Wade, R. (2009) 'From global imbalances to global reorganisations', *Cambridge Journal of
Economics*, 33(4), pp. 539–562. Available at: https://doi.org/10.1093/cje/bep032

White, S.K. (2012) 'Public health at a crossroads: assessing teaching on economic globalization as a social determinant of health', *Critical Public Health*, 22(3), pp. 281–295.
Available at: https://doi.org/10.1080 /09581596.2012.685052

Whoriskey, P., MacMillan, D. and O'Connell, J. (2020) ' "Doomed to fail": why a $4 trillion
bailout couldn't revive the American economy', *Washington Post*, 5 October. Available
at: www.washingtonpost.com /graphics/2020/business/coronavirus-bailout-spending/

Wikipedia (2023) *List of largest pharmaceutical settlements*. Available at: https://en.wikipe
dia.org/wiki/List_of_largest_pharmaceutical_settlements (Accessed: 7 February 2023).

Williams, S.N. and Nestle, M. (2015) '"Big Food": taking a critical perspective on a global
public health problem', *Critical Public Health*, 25(3), pp. 245–247. Available at: https://
doi.org/10.1080 /09581596.2015.1021298

Wood, B. *et al.* (2023) 'The double burden of maldistribution: a descriptive analysis of
corporate wealth and income distribution in four unhealthy commodity industries',
Critical Public Health, 33(2), pp. 135–147. Available at: https://doi.org/10.1080/09581
596.2021.2019681

Worldometer (2023) 'COVID-19 coronavirus pandemic'. Available at: www.worldometers.
info /coronavirus/ (Accessed: 7 February 2023).

7 Global health governance, the state, and healthy social movement activism

The previous chapter questioned whether our systems of governance could ensure a fair and healthy future. If we consider the 'polycrisis' we now confront, a neologism describing the conflux of persisting inequalities, climate chaos, biodiversity loss, rising illiberalism, and geopolitical conflict, it would be hard to conclude that it has But interrogating the reasons why remains important: as members of the 2014 *Lancet Commission on Global Governance for Health* concluded, because the "major drivers of ill health lie beyond the control of national governments and, in many instances, also outside of the health sector, we assert that some of the root causes of health inequity must be addressed within global governance processes" (Ottersen et al. 2014, p. 631). Governance is not the same as *government* (elected or otherwise), which remains the prerogative of nation-states and includes the singular right to use force. *Governance*, instead, refers to the messy and proliferating array of multistakeholder forums that involve governments and non-state actors in efforts to promote collective actions to achieve agreed-upon goals. Unlike government with its legislative and policing powers, governance actions are only rarely backed by formal authority structures.

Governance becomes more complicated at the global scale, as there is no institutional structure that resembles Westphalian nation-states and their governments. Global governance thus requires a high degree of collaboration amongst many different governments and non-state actors, with their competing agendas, in what has become an increasingly crowded space. The United Nations' various agencies alone number 38 distinct funding programmes, specialized agencies, adjoining entities, and related organizations. Although these are predominantly intergovernmental forums, they also frequently, and increasingly, include participation from corporate, philanthropic, and civil society organizations. The World Health Organization (WHO) is considered central to global governance (although see the Conclusion chapter for our remarks on the rapidly unfolding global political economic context at the time of writing) for health, but as Frenk and Moon (2013) noted a decade ago:

> There are now more than 175 [global health] initiatives, funds, agencies, and donors. To make matters even more complex, health is increasingly influenced

DOI: 10.4324/9781003654650-8

by decisions that are made in other global policymaking arenas, such as those governing international trade, migration, and the environment.

(p. 937)

Unsurprisingly, this messy melange of global health actors raises critical public health concerns around the structure, function, and power relations that inhere within governance systems. Many global health governance (GHG) platforms are public–private partnerships in which there is an assumed lack of conflict between for-profit entities and public health goals. Private sector actors in such partnerships usually outnumber those representing civil society interests. Most of these platforms, moreover, focus primarily on healthcare access issues and are often restricted to concerns with how to finance healthcare systems, thus largely omitting the role of socio-economic and environmental determinants of health. As Lee (2010) noted in a reflection on the release of the final report of the WHO Commission on Social Determinants of Health (CSDH):

> In a world increasingly influenced by non-state actors, and the coagulation of interests and distribution of power, authority and resources in ways that cut across, undermine, and even disregard state boundaries, is the strengthening of existing state-based institutions the only way forward? The transition from state-based to global institutions lies at the heart of current debates about GHG [global health governance] – how should political power be organised and exercised in a complex world crisscrossed by new constituencies not necessarily conforming to territorial states? ... Most problematically, perhaps, is how far WHO is capable of championing health equity given its diminished status in GHG. Political leverage depends on WHO having a leadership role in global health policy making.

(p. 13)

This chapter begins by asking whether we have coherence in governments' foreign policies that determine (or at least influence) the GHG domain or if such coherence is ever possible. It then examines the dominating influence of private economic interests in global governance for health before turning to how the COVID-19 pandemic opened up new veins for corporate profiteering while exacerbating economic inequalities and challenging public health prevention and control measures. It next discusses the One Health approach and the concomitant rise in antimicrobial resistance (AMR); that discussion sets the stage for an exploration of the different modalities (hard law/soft law) of GHG. It concludes with a discussion of the challenges our current global health era presents for progressive civil society activism.

Questioning policy coherence

Although policy incoherence is a routine political concern for governance at national and sub-national scales (witness how market-friendly financial policies often undermine citizen-friendly social protection policies), this lack of coherence also applies at global scales. As noted in the previous chapter, examples include trade and investment treaties empowering corporate over public good interests and neoliberal austerity policies disproportionately benefiting wealthier countries and citizens at the cost of adequately financed health systems for the world's poor. Anderson (2006) adds to these critiques a harsh assessment of the 'pro-poor health approach' of the health and development guidelines prepared by the Organization for Economic Cooperation and Development (OECD), the 'club' of rich countries, and the international forum advising most of the world's donor nations. Anderson argues that this approach, based on earlier World Bank (WB) and International Monetary Fund (IMF) structural adjustment (however much these have become nuanced in recent years in response to robust criticism), "is invariably one that facilitates entry of private for-profit investment, usually in the name of 'broad-based growth'" (p. 246). The OECD is not alone in advancing such 'privatization by stealth' that public health activist scholars have been challenging since at least the mid-1990s (Pollock 1995). Within a context of polycrisis, global governance platforms are increasingly attempting to leverage the (comparatively small) amounts of public financing proffered by governments to attract private investment funds. A recent analysis of this pro-private and market-friendly approach describes this as 'The Great Takeover' by corporations of global governance (People's Working Group on Multistakeholderism 2022).

Anderson (2006) goes on to point out how health development aid generally assumes that a simple expansion of financial resources will resolve any difficulties in health care access. Funding certainly helps, but if it comes with obligations to open financing and provision to private for-profit actors, however gilded with the market mantra of consumer choice, it does little to build an integrated public system or provide any guarantee of equitable access. This continues to play out in how the comprehensive model of Primary Health Care (first articulated in the 1978 Alma Ata Declaration, replete with its call for a socially just 'New International Economic Order') was displaced by universal health coverage, in which access to a limited list of healthcare services devolves to concerns of over insurance schemes (Labonté and Bodini 2022, Chap. B1; Sanders et al. 2019). The OECD guidelines further confound development assistance for water and sanitation systems by calling for "clearer recognition of the potential role of the private sector" (Organization for Economic Cooperation and Development 2003, p. 60). This, Anderson argues, presents unresolved interest conflicts, something few critical public health scholars would disagree with.

Development assistance, the focus of Anderson's (2006) contribution, is just one channel by which the foreign policies of nation-states rise up to become the normative or institutional frameworks for governing global health. Labonté (2008) identified at least five different foreign policy framings of health, which we expand on below: as security, as development, as global public good, as human right, and as commodity. The five foreign policy frames (also described as discourses) hold certain assumptions about how and why governments and global governance platforms should engage in collective health actions, with implications for how equitable those actions might be.

The most frequently cited frame, the *securitization of health*, is considered now to be a permanent feature of public health governance in the 21st century (Fidler 2007), and with SARS, SARS-CoV-2, and the risk of new zoonotic pandemics, it is likely to remain so. It represents the 'high politics' of international relations, with nations primarily concerned with securing the safety of their own borders. This plays out in inequitable ways, with funding (nationally and globally) following the interests of wealthier nations (e.g. emerging infections and zoonotic diseases with pandemic potential) and not necessarily the health needs of a global population, namely primarily endemic diseases that disproportionately affect poorer, low-income countries.

Mwacalimba (2012) provides the example of Zambia's response to the threat of H5N1 avian influenza ('bird flu'), where international funding "led to a distortion of the pandemic response" (p. 391). Following outbreaks and human fatalities in China, H5N1 was declared a 'zoonosis of public health concern'. To prevent its spread from outside the South Asian region, 'at-risk' parts of the developing world were offered financial assistance to prevent and control risk in their own poultry industries. However, Zambia's 'backyard' poultry farming was viewed as much the same as Asia's industrialized poultry production, where zoonotic risk is much greater, resulting in interventions that were "inappropriate when weighed against … the country's wider trade, agricultural and health priorities" (p. 391). The human resources involved came at a cost to other priority health needs such as HIV, malaria, and maternal mortality. Mwacalimba notes (2012):

> More widely, the avian and pandemic influenza saga reinforced positions taken by the industrialised members of the international community post-SARS, where … the perceived ramifications actually emphasized low probability Western concerns (mainly Europe and North America) over the costs of control for less developed economies and the livelihoods of Asian subsistence poultry producers whose flocks were targeted for control.
>
> (p. 400)

As Mwacalimba concludes, "the politics of disease control requires a more coherent marriage between the justifying evidence and local priorities to meaningfully contribute to the global health agenda" (p. 401), a message that resonates with post-COVID-19 pandemic accord negotiations, expected to complete by late May 2025. Using the risk of cross-border spread of multiple drug-resistant tuberculosis (TB), Horner and colleagues (2013) similarly argue that "in the post 9/11 era, there has been a conflation between public health and 'national security' concerns" (p. 418), leading to border and within-country control regimes that quickly become new technologies of surveillance. In Zambia's case, it was 'backyard chickens'; in the TB example, it was 'diseased' others (migrants) who become foreign risks to the body politic.

The *development frame* fares little better. Despite its pivot from viewing economic development as a precursor to health to health being regarded as an essential investment in development (generally viewed as economic growth), it suffers from being a charity rather than entitlement model that is subject to the whims of donor nations or large philanthropies such as the Gates Foundation. The instrumental reasoning behind health as an investment leads to several problems, including funnelling health financing into vertical disease-based programmes with short-term achievable targets, disproportionately rewarding aid-recipient countries with the 'right' set of economic policies as deemed by funders and rendering the causes and prevention of poverty and disease a technical matter rather than a political choice (Labonté 2008). As one illustration, Africa, a continent with many countries long reliant on development assistance, continues to lose more annually in capital flight, mostly illicit repatriation of corporate profits from extractive industries that then get banked in offshore financial centres (the polite term for 'tax havens'), than it receives in aid (Labonté and Ruckert 2019).

There is a long history of critical debate on the international development model of poverty reduction and health improvement. Proponents argue that such aid, which is delivered largely via donor countries' official development assistance (ODA) transfers, constitutes partial restitution for centuries of colonial exploitation. Others, like Anderson (2006), see aid as a new form of coloniality in which market economics replaces the costlier business of direct foreign rule. This debate heated up considerably in the early 2000s when the UN General Assembly declared Millennium Development Goals (MDGs), intended "to ensure that globalization becomes a positive force for all the world's people" (United Nations 2000, Section I. Values and principles). (The goals were to be reached by 2015; they were not.) Some argued that the aid dependency of the world's poorest countries trapped them in a client relationship with wealthier countries (Moyo 2009). Others countered with strong supportive evidence that without health aid transfers poorer nations could not provide the basic infrastructure needed to come anywhere close to achieving the health targets of the MDGs (Sachs 2014). Labonté and Ruckert (2019), drawing on some of the findings of the Globalization Knowledge Network of the WHO CSDH, split the difference:

> … development assistance has made, and will continue to make, an important equalizing contribution to global health outcomes; but it is best regarded not as a solution as such to globalization's disequalizing propensities, but rather as one of many needed means by which economic resources become more equitably distributed across the global population.
>
> (p. 158)

This conclusion immediately draws attention to a continuous and perverse maldistribution of wealth flowing from poor to rich countries, one that worsened considerably in the neoliberal era. The United Nations Conference on Trade and Development (UNCTAD) analysed net financial flows between developing and developed countries between 2000 and 2017. They measured all forms of capital that entered 134 developing countries (primarily foreign investment, loans, and ODA) and how much returned to developed countries (primarily loan payments, profit repatriation, and illicit financial flows) (UNCTAD 2020). The annual amounts of financial resources going from poor to rich countries ranged between $700 billion USD and $1.2 trillion USD, exceeding by multiple times the average of $100 billion USD in ODA that developing countries received:

> … leaving many developing countries on a debt treadmill, financially exhausted. External resources are deemed necessary to fund development, but this in turn generates return flows of interest payments and profit remittances that have to be funded by the developing country and can outweigh any earnings flows.
>
> (p. 2)

Although not necessarily a fan of ODA, UNCTAD further attests that, measured against donor countries' unmet pledge of providing 0.7 per cent of their gross national income to developing countries over the 17 years of the study period, the club of rich countries was short $2.7 trillion USD in unfulfilled commitments.

Wintrup (2022), in an ethnographic study of a global health partnership between Zambia and the US-based Clinton Foundation, provides an example of some of the subtle ways in which aid can unintentionally undermine the capacities of recipient government's health ministries. The intent of the partnership was to introduce a new cadre of 5000 community health workers to serve in rural areas, but, over time, Foundation officials "came to believe that senior Zambian government actors had granted them the authority to implement the programme outside of the formal channels of the government health system" (p. 608). Unlike the more forceful coloniality of donors or philanthropies stipulating the exact criteria for receiving health aid, Wintrup sees the Zambian case as a subtle form of 'outsourcing sovereignty', in which Foundation staff had more time, money, and resources to oversee the programme than did government health staff. Whatever the beneficence of intent, the effect "undermined the capacity of the state and created greater fragmentation in rural healthcare provision" (p. 609). Wintrup believes that this outsourcing dynamic "may be more common in global health partnerships than anthropologists and social scientists have recognised" (p. 617), thus adding another layer of complexity to the array of accountability measures aid-recipient countries already face from their scores of individual donor countries or partnership funders (Labonté and Ruckert, 2019).[1]

Similarly, although for different reasons, external funding for a response to the tenth Ebola epidemic in Democratic Republic of Congo (DRC) during 2018–2020 created an "atmosphere of mistrust" between responders and communities and spawned a ubiquitous expression amongst villagers: "Ebola is a business" (Park et al. 2022, from the title). In their (similarly) ethnographic study, the researchers eschew the oft-cited claim in global health literature that such mistrust is due to ignorance, misinformation, or the spread of conspiracy theories. Instead, they find that the characterization of Ebola "as a business" arose from critical community knowledge of the history of colonial interventions and the suspicion that powerful actors (local elites, international organizations, foreign countries) were profiteering from the scale of funding entering the country (as much as $1 billion USD in Ebola funding entered DRC). In other words, their jingoism is a rational reflection on the history of war, exploitation, and capital flight/impoverishment associated with the extractions of natural resources. As one interviewee commented on the meaning of the expression:

> It's not the population, there are some actors in the response who are misbehaving. We have the impression that they don't want the disease to be eradicated, because they make a lot of money.
>
> (p. 5)

The commonly encountered discrepancy between what non-local (international) health aid workers are paid compared to local health staff, which is sometimes as much as six-fold, adds to the financialized mistrust, with the "inhabitants of North Kivu and Ituri [the center of the Ebola outbreak] wonder[ing] why the response was not hiring people locally" (p. 6). Once mistrust supplants trust, it is hard for trust to be recuperated. In the Ebola instance, security forces were sent to communities to protect the 'responders', yet those same forces had routinely failed to protect communities from armed conflicts associated with first-world demand-generated extractivism.

The *global public goods discourse*, vaunted initially by economists working with the UN Development Programme, is seen by some as a tonic to the neocolonialism inherent in the charitable undertow of the development frame (Kaul et al. 2003). The global public goods concept is an expansion of utilitarian arguments for protecting public goods, meaning those that are open to all and non-exhaustible in use, that are subject to market failures arising from moral hazard (where the anticipation that governments will bail out disasters leads to failure to protect against risk of disaster in the first place) and 'free-riders' (where those who enjoy a benefit pay nothing for it). The post-2015 flurry of international agreements related to climate change, biodiversity, and the Sustainable Development Goals (SDGs), and the pledges to global funding platforms to address the agreements' commitments represent actions to protect the global public good of a biosphere supportive of human life, although the concept of public goods is itself rarely referenced. By contrast, *human rights*, with their panoply of covenants binding on those states that have ratified them, have more prominence in public health advocacy at both national and global scales. This is especially true when rights covenants are domesticated in national legislation, becoming justiciable using national courts (Gagnon and Labonté 2011). While invoked as a health foreign policy goal at least as often as is the development frame, the rights frame nonetheless falls well behind the top-ranked security and commodity frames (Ruckert et al. 2016; health as commodity in the context of trade was discussed in the previous chapter), both of which position economic interests above those of health and well-being.

Labonté's discussion of these overlapping but far from coherent frames was intended to aid public health advocates at the national scale in shifting governments' foreign policy in a healthier and more equitable direction. Drawing on moral philosophy, he further argues that government actors are moral actors, and they need to be challenged to make explicit their moral reasoning in deciding health and foreign policy priorities. But, as Labonté concludes (2008):

> A moral language ... is insufficient in itself as a global health discourse. Legal language is also needed and remains best provided in human rights covenants. Neither moral nor legal discourse (in the absence of enforcement mechanisms) is necessarily compelling as an economic or political rationale. Economically, both the global public goods and development discourses have some utility in policy debates, but only if they are located beneath a penumbra of ethical reasoning and legal obligation. Otherwise the risk exists that these discourses will lead to a triaging of foreign policy or global governance decisions that reflect the interests of wealthier nations.
>
> (pp. 478–479)

Politically, the security discourse is the most potent but remains the most problematic.

It may not be possible to avoid incoherence in foreign health policy anymore so than in domestic health policy. As Offe (1984) describes, this incoherence arises from the contradictory positioning of the state between markets and capital accumulation on the one hand and welfare provision for citizen/electorates on the other, which creates unresolvable legitimacy crises. Although Offe argues against socialist notions that the state can be 'occupied', he emphasizes that it can be 'used' by social movement groups to advance actions on their demands (more on this later in this chapter). Careful attention to invoking different health and foreign policy frames according to audience and strategic intent, as Labonté suggests, could help in such policy 'nudging' actions, albeit always with reference to the health equity implications of whatever foreign policy prerogative is chosen.

The dominating influence of private interests

One of the most important concerns with the state of GHG for critical public health research is the extent to which corporations have come to dominate the global market economy and in turn to sway governance (and government) decision-making away from social movement health equity demands. In 2018, 69 of the world's 100 richest entities were transnational corporations (Global Justice Now 2018). The value of the top ten corporations alone exceeded that of the world's bottom 180 countries (Accountancy Daily 2016). At the time of writing (early 2025), the disequalizing degree of private and public wealth and power has certainly tipped further to the corporate side of the (in)justice scales (Labonté and Ruckert 2019) (see also the Conclusion chapter of this volume). And, as Green (2019) noted, "public health has increasingly become the business of big (and small) business" (p. 357). This was seen in earlier chapters, including Chapter 6's discussion of the role of business (usually big) in promoting unhealthy commodities, often seeking collusion with public health authorities. Green offers some familiar examples: Public Health England joining up with the alcohol industry in an advertising campaign to promote alcohol reduction ('responsible drinking') as if a for-profit industry would be keen to reduce consumption or working with tobacco companies on ostensibly less-risky alternatives to smoking ('harm reduction') by supporting nicotine-addictive vaping. In Mexico, efforts in 2013 to impose a sugar tax on soda drinks were opposed by the country's health secretary and the medical director of the Mexican Diabetes Foundation, both of whom received industry funding to promote physical activity[2] (Labonté and Ruckert 2019). In 2010, a non-profit US-based foundation partnered with KFC to promote pink-hued buckets of fried chicken to raise funds for breast cancer awareness campaigns, despite evidence that overconsumption of such food could increase cancer risk (Anderssen 2010). In the same year, UNICEF-Canada partnered with the candy maker, Cadbury Adams Canada, that, in exchange for a half-million-dollar donation, pasted the respected UNICEF logo on all of its product packaging (Collier 2010).

Variously critiqued for its 'pink-', 'sugar-', or '(fill-in-the-blank)-washing', this well-known corporate marketing strategy takes on more subtle form when it is hidden behind the veil of philanthropy. As Green (2019) describes:

> *The Daily Mile* is a popular scheme in the UK to get primary school children running for 15 minutes each day in school time. It was started by a head teacher in Scotland and supported by a charity which promotes the scheme: a charity now entirely funded by INEOS, a large oil, gas, and petrochemicals company.
>
> (p. 257)

Powell (2014) expresses the same caution in his study of two obesity-prevention programmes involving partnerships between philanthropies, the food and drinks industry, and public or civil society organizations.[3] Corporate engagement is extensive, and it is promoted as being important to the obesity solution despite much public health research finding their business practices to be part of the obesity problem. As Powell argues, the public health concern may be less with the specific content of the educational programmes produced by such partnerships than with their neoliberal framing of the problem, which shifts responsibility away from corporations and towards individuals, a point remarked upon in earlier chapters of this volume. Anodyne education programmes with 'socially responsible' corporate branding, like UNICEF-monikered candies, help to deflect policy attention away from regulatory actions governing the industry. The message is that individuals, instead, must govern themselves. As Powell concludes, this "represents a noteworthy transformation in contemporary governance: The state's responsibility for the health, wealth, and education of the population has shifted to 'others' (corporations, charities, individuals)" (p. 234). As such, and as Green argues, public health concerns must now "go well beyond the potential moral taint of colluding with 'harmful commodity' industries" and focus more on the "growing, and under-researched, role of the private sector in general" (p. 258).

Baum, a frequent contributor to *Critical Public Health* and an Editorial Board member, has been leading a research group examining this lacuna over the past few years. Adopting methods now widely used in environmental, social, and HIAs, some of which are described in earlier chapters, this research group first articulated key elements of a 'corporate health impact assessment' by developing a framework for the many components at differing scales (Figure 7.1) (Baum et al. 2016).

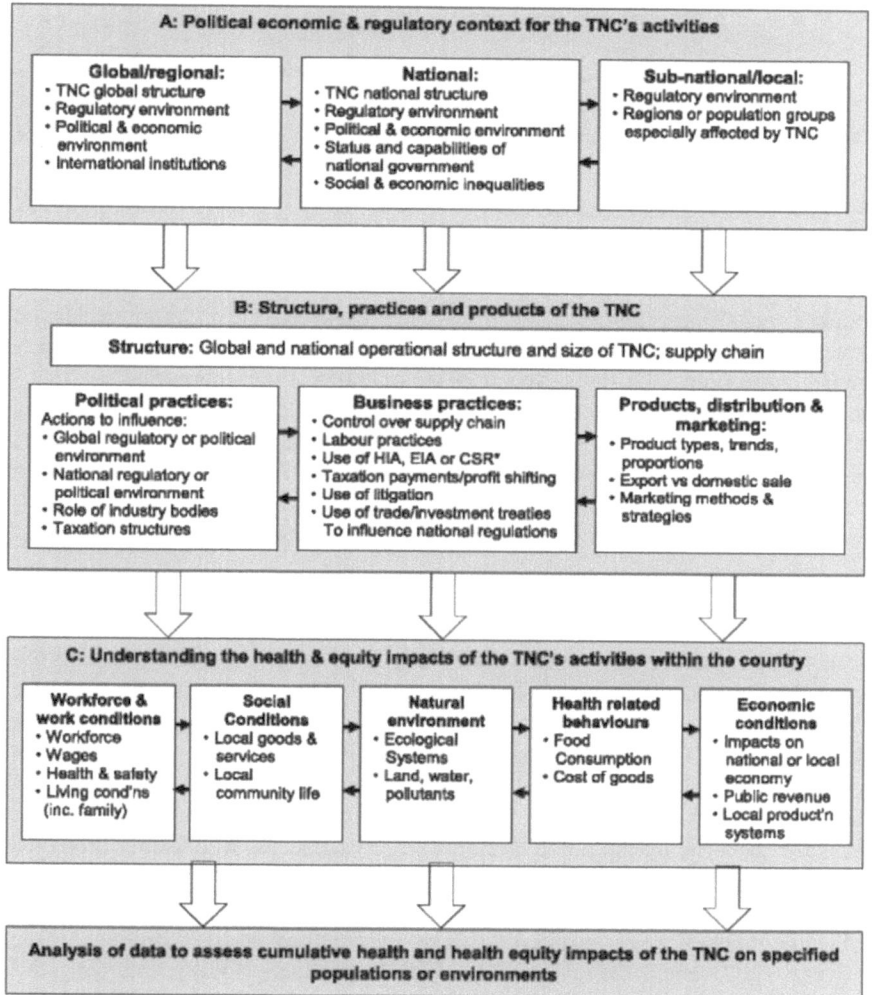

*HIA: Health Impact Assessment   EIA: Environmental Impact Assessment   CSR: Corporate Social Responsibility

Figure 7.1 A conceptual framework for conducting health impact assessments of corporations.

The intent was to apply the framework in studies of two sectors (food/beverages and extractives) with well-established health concerns. The framework was then tested empirically in a study of McDonald's Australia, using data drawn from documents, corporate literature, media items, and semi-structured interviews (Anaf et al. 2017). The results discussed both positive and negative health impacts. The main positive health outcome was "McDonald's investment in high levels of employment and training, and its inclusive, non-discriminatory workplaces" (p. 12/16), although this was somewhat outweighed by the sector's "lower wages and less secure conditions" (p. 13/16). These positive health benefits were further undermined by known or potential negative health impacts, arising from:

> … McDonald's ultra-processed food; its strategic industry alliances that facilitate corporate influence over food and advertising regulation; the loss of state revenue from its taxation strategies; and its health and environmental costs that are externalised to the community.
>
> (p. 12/16)

Notwithstanding acknowledged limitations in their assessment (e.g. no industry involvement in the study, no clear links between consumption of McDonald's products and chronic disease), the researchers regarded their Corporate Health Impact Assessment (CHIA) methodology to be a useful tool for civil society activists concerned with the health impacts of transnational corporate practices. They have since applied the same methodology, using similar data sources, to a study of the health impacts of a major extractive transnational (Rio Tinto) in its operations in Australia and South Africa (Anaf et al. 2022; Anaf et al. 2019) and an alcohol industry operating in Australia. They have identified similar mixed positive/negative impacts but an overall assessment tipping to the unhealthy side.

Enter the COVID-19 pandemic

The corporate market also wasted little time in finding new pathways to profit during the COVID-19 pandemic, most notably in the profiteering by the three pharmaceutical companies (Pfizer, BioNTech, and Moderna) responsible for the mRNA vaccines that dominated government vaccine purchases in 2020 and 2021. As many have pointed out, vaccine development was largely a result of investment and breakthroughs from publicly funded academic institutions with most of the financial risk borne by the public sector. The private sector was further protected from risk through advance purchase agreements and indemnification against legal action from adverse effects. All profits from vaccine sales went to the pharmaceutical companies. Pfizer profited the most, earning around $100 billion USD in two years (2021 and 2022) from its COVID-19 products (Erman and Wingrove 2023) reporting profits around 30 per cent (Macrotrends 2023), and paying just 7 per cent in taxes (CSI Market 2023) by availing itself of the many tax havens and transfer pricing chicanery afforded by liberalized global financial markets (Lalani et al. 2022). Both Pfizer and Moderna, along with other transnational corporations, fiercely opposed a 2021 intergovernmental agreement to raise minimum global corporate taxes to 15 per cent (Buntz 2021), a rate that most development economists argued should have been twice that. The extent of this profiteering is declining as the market for vaccines tapers off, but the lack of reform to laws protecting IPRs or public good requirements for government financing or assistance means the same inequitable system remains in place for when (not if) the next pandemic arrives. Suffice to say, as Speed et al. (2022) did, that COVID-19 "profiteering can be characterised as a policy failure of global pharmaceutical governance, where primacy (again) is given to economic rather than public health" (p. 45).

There are more subtle instances of the COVID-19 pandemic contributing to new forms of capital accumulation, such as Big Tech's sudden interest in contact tracing apps and how such apps can function as new platforms of 'surveillance capitalism' (Zuboff 2019). Zuboff regards this facet of tech-driven capitalism as an expansion of the collection of bio-behavioural data, the commercialized analysis of which is increasingly leveraged via machine learning and artificial intelligence (AI). French et al. (2022) analysed the Big Tech January 2020 rush to contact tracing app production through the lens of 'disaster capitalism', the term Klein (2007) earlier coined to describe the abilities of investors and entrepreneurs to transform human and environmental tragedies into cash machines (as wars have always done). The platforms owned by private capital and their use in 'data-mining' raise well-known privacy concerns, while the efficacy of these contact tracing apps (as with many new AI-driven apps) is subject to considerable debate regarding their "discriminatory design" and place in broader "algorithmic oppression" (French et al. 2022, p. 48). One critical issue with these contact tracing apps is that they are less concerned with helping cases seek treatment (if at all) or even to control contagion (see the previous chapter's discussion of 'faking global health' including a failed tech app attempt); rather, too often, they simply become a new form of policing, as demonstrated by a spatial analysis of racialized inequities in New York City police enforcement in the early months of COVID-19 mandates (Kajeepeta et al. 2022). The devices, the networks, the data storage, and the use of AI-enabled technology all work to "de-center the power of public health authorities" (French et al. 2022, p. 49) or, stated differently, to privatize such power. Marelli and colleagues (2022) regard this COVID-19 "techno-solutionism" as just another example of neoliberally tilted "responsibilization without contextualization" with its deployment:

> … premised on a perceived linear progression from science to applications to ethics, which entails delegating decisions about potentially sweeping social reconfigurations to innovation experts and scientists, with scant attention paid to the views, expectations, and normative-contextual stances articulated by publics and citizens.
>
> (p. 2).

That such apps failed to gain widespread public use or were proved ineffective does not detract from the need for ongoing critical examination of the health equity implications of ever more powerful and invasive forms of Big Tech's commercializing oversight of people's quotidian lives.

At a more macro-scale, the pandemic and its new infusion of wealthy countries' quantitative easing described in the previous chapter saw billionaire wealth zoom upwards, while most of the world's population experienced a drop in their incomes (Laborté 2022). The sudden appearance of a novel virus with lethal impact quickly drew mass attention to how some people fared much worse than others in both health and economic terms:

- The poor, the elderly, the racialized;
- The un/underhoused or informally settled;
- The undocumented or stateless migrants;
- The precariously (under-)employed;
- 'Essential' workers, health care or otherwise;
- Women whose domestic care work mushroomed;
- Those whose health was already compromised;
- Any of a number of other groups whose lives are characterized by social, economic, and political marginalization.

There is a growing body of critical public health literature on the intersectional inequities of these pandemic outcomes, such as the paper by Kapilashrami et al. (2022) documenting the ethnic disparities in health outcomes amongst health and social care workers engaged in COVID-19 care, a finding replicated in most other countries. Such studies are likely to continue as the world is not yet free of COVID-19 and not secure in terms of future zoonotic risks. As Speed et al. (2022) assert, continuing pandemic evaluations must "take into account the wider political contexts of public health action in determining which count as policy successes and which count as policy failures" (p. 1).

COVID-19 was not the first post-new millennial pandemic threat that challenged public health. Neither was it the first to be prone to controversy in countries' responses to its control, arising in part from what Leach et al. (2022) describe as 'incertitude' in the political management of knowledge. Almost a riff on former US defence secretary Donald Rumsfeld's 2002 post-9/11 comment about 'known knowns, known unknowns, and unknown unknowns' (Zak 2021), incertitude describes how as "disease and its social life unfold, 'potential uncertainties', constructed in future planning, may become actualised" (Leach et al. 2022, p. 84). The authors assess several recent pandemics for how the 'known unknowns' (uncertainties and ambiguities) played out in the complex messiness of people's lives, often distant from the calm assuredness of technocratic response planning. Echoing Parks et al. (2022), the refusal of Congolese peoples during the 2018–2020 Ebola outbreak in DRC to participate in contact tracing or vaccination arose from mistrust, with Leach et al. 2022 noting:

... citizens [wondering] why Ebola was prioritised over other health issues in an already limited health system. In turn, mistrust was exacerbated by the disruptive 'Ebola economy'; as resources and finance scaled up, so did contestation amongst already fragmented local political authorities. Thus, a new set of uncertainties and ambiguities unfolded in the dynamic relationship between local socio-politics and response activities.

(p. 85)

Interventions for intermittent Nipah outbreaks in South Asia (1998–2001), a less common but more lethal bat-transmitted disease, rarely attended to such co-factors as lack of basic hygiene, ambulances, medical supplies, and healthcare services, focusing instead on the development of vaccines and therapeutics with an "underlying assumption in the scientific community … that persistent scientific endeavour will ultimately resolve the ongoing uncertainties" (p. 86). The cholera outbreaks in Haiti (2010 and 2022) and Yemen (2016), complicated by disasters (earthquake, war) and occurring in the midst of humanitarian crises, questioned whether even the best-laid preparedness plans would have mattered. Leach et al. 2022 state:

> Unless preparedness practices – modelling, surveillance, stockpiling, administering treatments and so on – are deployed with a deeper understanding of context, with the real lives of those who are vulnerable to cholera at the centre, plans will fail; unravelling through a combination of inevitable ignorance, deep uncertainties about everything from the epidemiology to cultural behaviours and ambiguities over the origins of and reasons for outbreaks.

(p. 88)

'Incertitude' certainly characterized the two early years of COVID-19. Some thought the pandemic marked one of public health's finest hours, but as the assessments of policy successes and failures continued to roll in, what became striking was the range of differences in how public health authorities responded from episodic lockdowns to laissez-faire voluntarism to often punitive zero-COVID extremes. One commonality was the hesitancy for public health authorities, from the WHO downwards, to acknowledge openly the degree of uncertainty, as if the populace would be unable to accept any ambiguity in messaging. As Leach et al. (2022) caution, disease preparedness thinking must move "beyond resource investment and system strengthening" with its "reliance on models, predictions and control-oriented solutions" to "alternative, open-ended methodologies that embrace uncertainty" and in which "socially-just and ethical preparedness plans … emerge through dialogue and deliberation" (p. 93).

One Health and the rise of antimicrobial resistance

In tandem with the increase in zoonoses, what became known as a One Health approach began to capture global health attention. Conceptually, this approach focuses on how interactions between humans, animals, and the environment can enhance health or create disease risk. Although it is a relatively new term, One Health's underlying analysis predates industrialization and draws from traditional or Indigenous health knowledge systems (Mumford et al. 2023). Until recently, it confined most of its attention to the human/animal interface with an emphasis on surveillance-response and an anthropocentric legacy that positioned human health above that of most animals. The centrality of the environment was recognized but given short shrift by three international organizations (World Health Organization (WHO), Food and Agriculture Organization, and World Organization for Animal Health) which formalized a global One Health collaboration in 2010. In 2022, the tripartite was joined by the United Nations Environment Programme (UNEP), thus forming a novel quadripartite governance structure. The quadripartite's new and expansive understanding of One Health is said to go "way beyond emerging infections and novel pathogens; it is the foundation for understanding and addressing the most existential threats to societies, including AMR, food and nutrition insecurity, and climate change" (The Lancet 2023, p. 169). The related concepts of EcoHealth (bringing a more systems-based approach) and planetary health (with its emphasis on our ecocidal threats) help to address the loss of the ecologic focus that was One Health's initial base. There remain, however, a few caveats, as Green (2012) cautioned early on in the concept's global rise:

> If … a One Health perspective is a reminder that a fully ecological approach to public health needs to take our relations with other species into account, a critical perspective is also a corrective to assuming that those ecologies are in any way natural systems, comprehensible as if they existed outside the discourses that bring them into being. A second implication of thinking about One Health from a critical perspective is that we also need to be critical of the categories of 'disease' that are prioritised within the interfaces between animal and human health. An overly medicalised model of risks in terms of infectious (zoonotic) disease leaves insufficient space for a consideration of social wellbeing, and how this might be mediated in terms of relations with other species.
>
> (p. 379)

Other critiques of One Health include its neglect of the critical political economy perspective identified by both Green (2012) and Mwacalimba (2012). One Health's most recent call for "greater, more proactive investment in preventive interventions, and in integrating surveillance–response in environmental, animal, and human systems" (Zinsstag et al. 2023, p. 592) may bring more planetary health into the calculi but does not overcome the political silence. As Green (2012) wrote:

> … a critical perspective is a reminder that we cannot treat systems of animal, human and environmental interrelationships as purely natural phenomena, which create, transform or manage infectious disease risk. Those networks are brought into being materially by political systems, such as the forces of globalization … and … discursive framings, which make some risks more visible than others, and some populations more liable to intervention as legitimate objects of public health surveillance than others.
>
> (p. 380)

What has been called the 'slow burn' of AMR (in contrast to the rapid spread of pandemics) will almost certainly keep the One Health approach high in GHG's pantheon. The two are entwined, with the global COVID-19 pandemic leading to more antibiotic use and speeding up the risk of AMR (Nature Microbiology 2020). Blame (and hence remedy) for AMR is apportioned by economic interest, as Glover et al. (2022) found in their critical discourse analysis of drug industry stakeholder submissions to a UK inquiry into AMR. Adopting a 'policy dystopia model' that asserts that "interested parties (typically industry) will argue that policies disadvantageous to their interests will lead to a dystopian future including widespread adverse economic, political, and social effects" (p. 4), the researchers revealed how industry submissions argued their self-interest in paradoxical ways. These included urging offers of subsidies and incentives to themselves but avoiding any regulations; extolling the power of their industry in already dealing with AMR via its investments, but simultaneously pleading powerlessness to influence drug misuse by others; and lauding the value of their for-profit model while also bragging about their not-for-profit work. The well-worn corporate strategic playbook was in play, including coordination, in the form of cross-referencing their submissions, using the same arguments, and crowding out the more diverse submissions from civil society; and blame-shifting, by shifting the narrative from a focus on drugs to one on diagnostics, from human use to animal misuse and from industry accountability to individual responsibility.

Rejecting both the individual behaviour change and pump-priming new discovery approaches that have characterized policy response to AMR, Broom and colleagues (2022) draw on a decade of qualitative interviews with clinicians in Australia, UK, and India, to reframe AMR as a social and political concern that results from a confluence of factors and practices. They describe these as temporal myopia (short-termism, not seeing long-term impacts with an emphasis on short-term management); individualization (with a focus on individual practitioner behaviours, reinforced by Western rationality generally and neoliberal ideology more specifically); marketization (the pursuit of profitable monopoly rights for products of interest in HIC markets); and human exceptionalism, in which actions on AMR devolve to actions protecting human (but not animal or environmental) health. Missing in AMR policy, they contend, is a proper analysis of its social determination; instead, AMR is regarded as an exogenous threat rather than as a continuing anthropogenic creation. To counter this, the authors call for "solidaristic models that espouse collective responsibility and recognise relative opportunity to act" (p.451), while drawing attention to how structural inequalities underlying much human misuse:

> coupled with the global mobility of resistant genes and bugs, speaks to the importance of cultivating globally solidaristic models to counter AMR. Such an approach would recognise shared vulnerability alongside disproportionate capacity to act, ideally fostering a willingness among those well positioned to act to accept some of the 'costs' of local action.
>
> (p. 460)

In a later contribution, Broom et al. (2023) unpack the concept of AMR vulnerability, dismissing the "individual (mis)behaviour" (of people, clinicians, farmers which creates vulnerability) and invoking "critical social science" that routinely offers "fundamentally structural account of vulnerability that foregrounds the evolving and agentic ways vulnerability is produced through the (historical and present-day) social, political, economic and environmental organisation of life" (p. 3). In reviewing this literature, the authors distinguish between a number of different AMR vulnerabilities: *embodied*, meaning how the contexts in which people are born create a 'microbial vulnerability' that can be transmitted intergenerationally; *assembled*, referring to how the dynamics of AMR vulnerability change through social processes that can enhance microbial vulnerability and the institutions, industrial, and market systems that lead to misuse and hence to AMR itself; *intersectional*, in which co-morbidities, social stigma, and multiple axes of inequality reinforce embodied and assembled vulnerabilities; and *surveillance* which, in the absence of explicating social contexts, can paradoxically increase rather than decrease biological AMR vulnerability. Broom et al. (2023) note:

> Such a critical conception of vulnerability has the potential to help attune (emerging and evolving) AMR solutions towards a focus on systematic vulnerability, which recognises bodies as articulations of the nexus of biology, culture, ecologies and economic conditions. Vulnerability is the underlying issue to be addressed, and not simply the context for intervention.
>
> (p. 8)

Global health governance: hard law or soft law?

Both the pandemic and AMR have accelerated debates about not only how GHG is constituted (e.g. to what extent should civil society, corporate, or philanthropic interests be engaged, and how?) but also what form such governance should take. Magnussen and Patterson (2021) address this with a focus on noncommunicable diseases (NCDs) and the impact different global governance modalities are likely to have on national government policies and regulations. Their legal review identified four distinct governance forms:

1 Global normative and legal instruments ('soft law' instruments such as agreements on global strategies, plans of action, codes of practice, and guidelines; and 'hard law' treaties and conventions);
2 Political accountability mechanisms (goals, targets, indicators, and timelines such as those found in the SDGs, but also 'shadow reports' and measures developed by civil society organizations);
3 Provision of development assistance (financial assistance to entice or loan conditionalities to enforce certain national-level policy changes);
4 Purpose-build governance mechanisms (incorporating any or all of the above forms but within the multistakeholder governance platforms that have come to dominate much GHG).

The WHO is prolific in creating normative (non-binding) instruments which, as the authors point out, can impact national policies:

> ... not only because of the persuasive force of these documents, or their formal status, but because of the political processes that precede their development. The World Health Assembly and UN General Assembly are global political forums that provide opportunities for debate, for receiving evidence, generating consensus and exerting political pressure on Member States.
>
> (p. 468)

Some of these normative instruments may include indicator checklists, but, unlike treaties, there are no legal obligations for compliance by member states. The 'soft law' national action plan on NCDs (2013–2020) and its 2017 appendix of 'best buys', while non-binding, nonetheless emphasize legal and regulatory change, costly endeavours for many low-income countries (LICs) facing huge resource capacity issues, a recurring issue in all forms of GHG. The WHO Constitution provides the World Health Assembly with the authority to enact legally binding conventions or agreements within any topic area of WHO competence. To date, only two such 'hard law' treaties have been agreed upon: the 2003 Framework Convention on Tobacco Control (FCTC), ratified by 182 countries (World Health Organization 2023a), and the International Health Regulations (IHRs), binding on all 196 member states[4] (World Health Organization 2023b). Lobbying by tobacco transnationals and the poverty reduction narrative of tobacco farming, which we critically discussed in Chapter 6, has made it difficult for some countries to domesticate in national legislation the FCTC's binding protocol requirements. Nonetheless, the convention's existence has prompted calls for the WHO to negotiate other binding treaties, including on global health, on alcohol, and on obesity and healthy diets. As Magnusson and Patterson (2021) note:

> The existence of such conventions could impose additional pressures on countries that assumed obligations under them to implement these global standards through national laws and policies. On the other hand, legally-binding instruments are time consuming to negotiate and are products of a political process: to the extent that they embody weak or unduly flexible standards, they might achieve little in real terms.
>
> (p. 467)

Even then, the question of enforcement remains. Apart from political pressure from other nations or the public 'naming and shaming' of failing to fulfil treaty obligations, there is little that the WHO or any other UN or affiliated intergovernmental organization can do to enforce compliance. The most powerful global treaties are considered to be those governing trade and finance where there is "considerable and consistent evidence of intended effects" (Hoffman et al. 2022, p. 5), which is attributed to the costs involved in countries' non-compliance:

For treaties governing environmental, human rights, humanitarian, maritime, and security policy domains, the only modifiable treaty design choice with the potential to improve effectiveness appears to be the inclusion of enforcement mechanisms.[5]

(p.5)

Ruckert et al. (2020) tackled this issue of compliance and enforcement with respect to AMR in a narrative review of global governance mechanisms. As per Magnussen and Patterson (2021), they placed such mechanisms in one of two categories: binding or non-binding. A binding treaty is considered the 'gold standard' in global governance. None presently exists for AMR, but if it were negotiated, it would likely improve reporting and accountability, create obligations for surveillance, prevent market and competitive disadvantages for countries complying with stewardship requirements while others are not, and even proscribe marketing of antimicrobials as part of a conservation strategy. The challenge in achieving such an agreement is probable opposition by domestic stakeholders, largely agricultural industries. Legally binding regulations focusing only on antimicrobial use may be easier to achieve. At present, the peak global statement on AMR governance is the non-binding 2015 AMR Global Action Plan (World Health Organization 2015) which lacks "effective mechanisms for transparency, oversight, and complaint, providing little international pressure or incentives for countries to comply with the unenforceable terms" (Ruckert et al. 2020, p. 520). Just before COVID-19's arrival, the One Health tripartite (WHO, OIE, WOAH) envisioned an intergovernmental treaty or multistakeholder AMR Protocol by 2030; the pandemic then incentivized this aim, including revisions to the IHRs (which were agreed upon during the 2024 World Health Assembly) or via a new pandemic accord in final negotiation with a hopeful signing date of May 2025. The AMR governance review, while critical, concludes with an equivocation:

Deep and divergent perspectives remain (often implicit rather than explicitly stated) about the causal relation between legal and normative change:

- Is norm change a necessary antecedent to generating the political will required to produce legal change in the form of a binding agreement?
- Or does legal change, by compelling changes in actors' behaviour and policies, represent the catalyst for a subsequent change in reinforcing norms? (p. 524).

The pandemic has placed this equivocation under politically charged global scrutiny. The ignominious experience of vaccine hoarding and profiteering[6] alongside WHO efforts to counter the decline in its assessed contributions and concerns over a drop in its public trust (Guo et al. 2022) created the context in which two parallel WHO governance negotiations are underway: revisions to the IHRs and creation of a new pandemic accord. Both negotiations, like the pandemic itself, reveal deep-seated differences between developed and developing countries that revolve around equity and financial inequalities (Patnaik 2023a). At the IHR negotiating table, developing country amendments focused on equity and financing, while wealthy nations were more interested in amendments to strengthen obligations on compliance and information sharing (Patnaik 2023b). Around the pandemic accord negotiating table, unenforceable 'soft law' preambular nods in the direction of equity abound, with 'hard law' language reserved for emphases on security and surveillance (Third World Network 2023). Dividing lines persist around reforms to IPRs (given the failure of the Trade-Related Aspects of Intellectual Property Rights (TRIPS) waiver to achieve what its proponents had intended) and benefit-sharing obligations in return for developing country pathogen-sharing. Developing countries have been demanding enforceable binding commitments of financial support and vaccine access in the accord articles covering 'pathogen access and benefit sharing'; high-income countries have yet to yield to these demands (as of March 2025).

These are not new contentions. From a critical public health vantage, the outcomes of these negotiations must reduce the financial and political power differentials within and between nations and strengthen accountable public governance over that of private influence in multistakeholder platforms.[7] To that end, there is a growing number of activist public health researchers joining with civil society organizations to press for such reforms at national government levels and, when allowed, in consultations with the intergovernmental negotiating forums.

The civil society challenge

Magnussen and Patterson (2021), in their somewhat dismal assessment of the state of national actions emanating from current approaches to the global governance of NCDs, call for a "more vigorous global social movement ... framed in terms to health justice, to press governments for greater accountability and global donors for greater resources" (p. 473). The same holds true for our current moments in GHG, with the treaty and IHRs being only one instance with trade and investment treaty reforms. Overhauling the Bretton Woods institutions, and enforcing measures to avoid climate collapse and ecocide, comprise a few prominent others.

It's useful to start a discussion of civil society/social movement activism by digging a bit further back in the pages of *Critical Public Health*. In a 2006 paper, Scambler and Kelleher (2006) discuss the advocacy potential of new social movements (NSM), a term that began its sociological ascendency in the 1990s and which they describe as collective resistance to neoliberal capital accumulation and 'hyper'-commodification. NSM theory arose in distinction from the then-dominant (and largely North American-based) 'resource mobilization theory' of collective action, which emphasized the importance of formalized social movement organizations that aimed to gain recognition as legitimate political actors and to increase material benefit (resources) going to those represented by the movement (Cohen 1985). NSM theorists argued that, rather than simply pursuing interests through forming bureaucratic organizations, social movements are primarily cultural expressions against dominant ways of viewing society and social relations. They are counter-hegemonic formations, engaged in conflict over ideas and not simply (or at all) over material resources or actual decision-making authority. Collective action can be expressed politically (demonstrations against the state, lobbying, and so on), but the political goals of social movements are self-limiting. While accepting the importance of class-based social movements, Scambler and Kelleher identify an overlapping typology of NSMs in the public health space with different mobilizing potentials: rights-based activism, self-help groups, campaigns, identity, and political struggles. In current forms, we might identify some of these as, respectively, LGBTQ++ and human rights; patient self-help and anti-privatization advocacy; networks lobbying against unhealthy commodities; Indigenous, anti-racist ('Black Lives Matter'), and transgender identity claims; and anti-globalization and environmental (e.g. extinction rebellion) mobilizations. As "organized foci for resistance" against the "economic liberalism and the reinvigoration of transnational corporate capitalism", the diversity of NSMs creates a more generalized "culture of challenge" (p. 229).

Lee et al. (2021) describe such a cultural challenge in their analysis of a 'Corporate Killing Movement' (CKM), a joint labour/civil society alliance that arose in South Korea in the early 2000s in response to vulnerable working conditions at the lower end of the labour pyramid that led to a high rate of workplace deaths. The movement's branding was unusual, given that the country was known for regarding its corporate conglomerates as almost sacred and essential to its modern globalized economy. The study used 'dialectical critical realism' and framing to explain the movement's origin and activism, regarding it as an exemplar of public health movement activism. Lee et al. (2021) note:

> In keeping with the critical realist approach in treating structure and agency as a mutually constitutive amalgam, our analysis focused on examining how workers' collective agency was constrained by existing social structures, and how collective agency emerged and evolved to transform constraining structures.
>
> (p. 158)

CKM's efforts to translate its activist claims into legislation failed, which the authors attribute to the absence of a strong pro-labour political party in the country. However, the attention their campaigning created was associated with improvements in health and safety enforcement.

The CKM article was part of a special issue of *Critical Public Health* on the theme of social movements and collective agency, which posed the question: "How is public health activism adapting to changing times, which often seem increasingly hostile to human rights and social justice claims?" (Campbell and Cornish 2021, p. 125). As also discussed in the Introduction chapter, the guest editors took an expansive view of collective agency as residing in "any activities by members of vulnerable groups and their allies that increase their opportunities for health and well-being" (p. 126). Peer education and community mobilization are seen as 'agentic' acts alongside social movements, whereas others would see the first two more as developmental precursors to the third, emphasizing the explicitly political intent (or challenge) of social movements (e.g. Labonté and Laverack

2008). Collective agency is seen as arising not just in the visible form of protests, sit-ins, demonstrations, and other acts of advocacy, but also in the direct care of marginalized persons (imparting esteem and value of health importance beyond the actual service being offered) and in 'below the radar' acts to redistribute resources to less privileged groups even when institutional norms may not allow it. These "microscopic processes", the guest editors argue, point to "new ways of thinking about the workings of power, the nature of the goals of health-enhancing collective action, and the processes and outcomes of public health activism" (p. 131). Critical public health, they suggest, needs to give more regard to collective action as processes and not just as outcomes, as being both explicit (externally visible) and implicit (more inter-relational, even invisible).

One example of process as activism describes the reclaiming of the Nhanga, in Shona/Bantu societies "a traditional round hut for girls and young women at a homestead" as a "cultural innovation to shift harmful social norms" (Gumbonzvanda et al. 2021, p. 170). Although superficially similar to the consciousness-raising groups of second-wave 1960s feminist praxis, the authors' work "attempts to decolonise the safe space knowledge base, positioning the Nhanga, and safe spaces more broadly, as a tactic originating within African cultural histories" (p. 171). Recognizing physical space as an important form of power, their collaborative autoethnographies describe the use of the Nhanga in different global, national, and community-level governing spaces as a tool that disrupts "expected installations of power" (p. 174). As described by the guest editors Campbell and Cornish (2021):

> Originally developed in Zimbabwe, the contemporary Nhanga is a form of quiet activism in small, informal anti-hierarchical spaces in which dominant power relations of gender and age are suspended, and all voices are given equal attention and value irrespective of social status. It strengthens 'emotional citizenry' through providing affective, narrative and cultural spaces that reveal the power, resourcefulness and creativity of young African women, a group often silenced in mainstream public spheres.
>
> (p. 129)

Bodini et al. (2020) in a multi-country study of civil society engagement under the PHM's campaign rubric of 'Health for All' (HFA) place "a premium on the subjectivity of activists rather than the objectivity of the researchers" (p. 387), a stance that resonates with the inter-relational dimensions of health activism. Using a participatory action research (PAR) design of repeat cycles of data collection and analysis, the researchers draw from multiple case studies, programme evaluations, and activist narratives, all undertaken with the explicit intent of informing ongoing health activist practice. A thematic analysis by Sanders et al. (2018) summarizes key activism principles under five core domains:

- Movement building (understanding pathways to activism);
- Campaigning and advocacy (the heart of social movement activism);
- Capacity building (formal but often learning by doing);

- Knowledge generation and use (critical assets in political struggles);
- Engaging with governance (policy dialogue with structural critique).[8]

One of the case studies in the larger research project involved in-depth interviews with fifteen health activists who shared a long history of social movement activism (Musolino et al. 2020), locating their narratives within a socio-political analysis of the global trends of late modern individualism and capitalist neoliberalism. One of these trends is how post-1990 civil society was "co-opted by governments and aid agencies" in which "debates about the economic role of civil society dominate over their cultural and political significance, especially as states continue to retreat from their social obligations to provide essential services" (p. 10). The interviewed activists underscored the importance of building and sustaining a political or ideological foundation for their work, something they found often lacking in formal nongovernmental organizations (NGOs) and the institutionalized 'resource mobilization' movements described earlier by Scambler and Kelleher (2006). This foundational commitment nonetheless created a campaigning dilemma: single issue or deep analysis? Musolino et al. 2020 note:

> The simple message of a particular issue is good grist for campaigning. But without being anchored in a deeper … statement on societal structures of power, it lacks the ability to build a broad-based civil society movement for the type of society that might transform the escalations in … inequalities.
>
> (p. 11)

This dilemma becomes more challenging when navigating the links between local and global advocacy efforts, with the "dangers of investing too heavily in either the global or local" (p. 11).

> Policy dialogue was seen to complement other forms of activism, such as working in community health clinics. There was, however, a caution raised of activists seeing community work as more 'authentic' than engaging in policy dialogue, especially at global scales [given that] the local and global are intrinsically connected in the current globalised era and thus, despite the challenges of globalisation, the struggle for health equity must work at all levels of society.
>
> (pp. 11–12)

The scalar quandary is not simply global/local, but also national (with global resonance) and geographically diffuse, as elaborated in a study of health workers' resistance struggles against austerity measures in two differing country contexts (Spain and the UK) (Ribera-Almandoz and Clua-Losada 2021). Described as a "White Tide" (*Marea Blanca*) in Spain, white-coated health workers took to the streets to protest the privatization of much of Spain's public health system in 2021. What began as a local protest in Spain quickly became a national movement. The same occurred in the UK, originating in Manchester in 2005 but then growing into a loosely networked series of groups opposing privatization. The main argument in this analysis of these two events is the importance of social movements engaging in multi-scalar organizing since, as the authors argue, drawing from both sociology and political geography, "scales are temporary and unstable spaces of conflict and compromise that offer significant avenues for disruptive resistance and emancipatory social change" (p. 183). Not only was there scaling up (from local initiatives to national protests allowing the "judicialisation of politics" through bringing court actions into campaign demands, much as is now happening in green activist movements, notably around climate change) and scaling down (where national protests motivate local actions with emphases on local coalition building, critical education moments, and physical sit-ins), but, in Spain, the *Marea Blanca* also joined with many other activist organizations in a more general campaign against austerity measures. Ribera-Almandoz and Clua-Losada (2021) note:

> On the one hand, they developed localised and territorially rooted forms of mobilisation, which have been useful means for the construction and strengthening of community relations by connecting workers, activists and neighbours through their everyday needs and demands, and have allowed for the experimentation with forms of grassroots organisation, collective deliberation, and horizontal decision making. On the other hand, the formation of trans-local networks of struggle contributed to the development of coordinated political actions, and of alternative collective narratives that effectively defied widespread official discourses.
>
> (p. 190)

There are many past and present accounts of successful social movement activism, whether or not under a 'health' umbrella, and the People's Health Movement (PHM) study emphasizes the importance of "know your history", a reference to "social movements' deep roots" (Bodini et al 2020, p. 392). But not all campaigns achieve their aims, thus surfacing one of the greatest barriers to sustained activism: despair in the face of continued failure. Cornish (2021) confronts this challenge in her analysis of the 'thwarted' activism following the 2019 Grenfell Tower fire in London, where her own despair at so little change despite the persistence of 'affected people turned activists' "met a counter-weight: The … persistence and boldness of survivors and bereaved families" (p. 294). Invoking Haraway's "relational ontology and particularly its central idea of 'staying with the trouble'" (p. 294), which sidesteps the hope/despair binary of activism, Cornish "explores the trajectories of six different [Grenfell] activist change efforts: a fire safety campaign, engagements with a public inquiry, campaigns to preserve community assets, community gardening, silent walks, and provision of support to children at a community centre, each addressing social determinants of health and 'staying with the trouble' in different ways" (p. 293). Two key precepts from her study stand out: Firstly, "catastrophic loss and destruction [such as the Grenfell Tower fire] are not separate to caring, hopeful projects, but co-present and implicated in creative caring efforts", a phenomenon almost universally recounted as sequelae to human tragedies; but, secondly, "hope must be enacted to be worthwhile" (p. 295). Even if those enactments 'fail' in some sense (she cites how a fire safety campaign was turned down by parliament), "in every effort before and after the bitter setback, care for human life is asserted, and a caring world is remade" (p. 303).

In other words, the critical elements of sustained social movement health activism can be distilled to caring for others and acting (in some fashion) on that care.

Notes

1 One of the authors recalls a research visit to a sub-Saharan African (SSA) country in the early 2000s, where most of the central health ministry's planning staff time was consumed with writing up reports to the scores of separate donor groups rather than health system planning. A representative of the country's largest donor was seconded to the office of the health minister to provide ongoing programme implementation oversight. Although the early 2000s' surge in new global health partnerships eventually slowed, it was more recently reinvigorated in response to COVID-19 and 'health security' concerns with future pandemic preparedness and response.

2 The 'energy out' physical activity is usually the first line of defence in the face of proposed regulatory measures aimed at reducing consumption of unhealthy commodities, notably sugary drinks. But there are discordant voices in the public health community regarding 'sin taxes', originally dating back to tobacco excise taxes (hardest on the poor, as are all consumption taxes). Increasingly, this line of argument is being applied to sugary drinks taxes, which are argued as creating 'weight-stigmatization' (Waugh et al. 2022) or unfairly targeting Indigenous communities (Tait and Riediger 2021). There are merits in such critiques, insofar as they identify the social and economic inequities that may underpin high intake of sugary drinks by poor or Indigenous populations. However, a singular focus on the tax alone, without interrogating the role of industry in creating high-sugar-content products, does little to reduce the disproportionate burden of disease associated with excess consumption of these products.

3 One of these civil society organizations, a Canadian-based programme, became defunct in 2017 "due to a decline in business" (Wikipedia n.d.), meaning its corporate members were no longer funding production of its signature public service announcements.

4 Not all WHO member states signed the FCTC; the USA did sign but has not ratified it and rarely accepts oversight by any international treaty. This includes the WTO whenever its independent dispute rulings go against its perceived national interests. Trump's 2025 US withdrawal from the WHO, described further in the Conclusion chapter, includes withdrawal from the IHR ratification and any pandemic accord negotiations or agreement.

5 It is important to recognize that most of the treaty evaluations in this study's meta-analysis concerned trade and finance treaties; only 2 of the 32 non-finance treaties had any enforcement measures, and there was no consideration of the counterfactual (what might have occurred in the absence of the treaties lacking enforcement measures but potentially carrying normative influence). Its caution regarding the importance of enforcement, however, has not gone unnoticed in discussions surrounding the new pandemic accord and IHR reforms, discussed below.

6 This practice continued with the 2022 Mpox outbreak in Africa. Despite affected countries requiring ten million vaccines, only one million were made available, while 99% were stockpiled in high-income countries. The vaccine manufacturer (Bavarian Nordic)

to date has refused to license the vaccine for low-cost generic manufacture elsewhere and charges ten times more per dose than estimates of the production costs for developing country manufacturers. Should 'bird flu' (H5N1, or avian influenza) spread more easily to humans (it is already manifesting a small number of cross-species human infections), the same scenario is likely to repeat, absent enforceable provisions in a new pandemic accord that are being demanded by developing countries. (Third World Network, open letter 17 February 2025.)

7 A wild card in the midst of these two already complex governance negotiations is discussion of creating a new public–private partnership under the WHO authority to deal with access and affordability of pandemic-related medicines to low- and lower-middle-income countries. This is in line with what Big Pharma has been lobbying for, as it would leave middle- and high-income countries open to profiteering on new drug, diagnostics, or vaccine discoveries.

8 A full report of the case studies and programme evaluations can be found here: https://phm ovement.org/cse4hfa/. A special supplement of the Brazilian journal, *Saúde em Debate* (January 2020), contains several articles based on the individual studies (in English, Spanish, or Portuguese) and can be found here: https://revista.saudeemdebate.org.br/sed/ issue/view/33/v.%2044%2C%20n.%20ESPECIAL%201.

References

Accountancy Daily (2016) 'Corporations dominate world's top 100 economic entities' *Business & Accountancy Daily*, 14 September, www.accountancydaily.co/corporations-dominate-worlds-top-100-economic-entities (Accessed: 10 February 2023).

Anaf, J. *et al.* (2017) 'Assessing the health impact of transnational corporations: a case study on McDonald's Australia', *Globalization and Health*, 13(7). Available at: https://doi.org/ 10.1186/s12992-016-0230-4

Anaf, J. *et al.* (2019) 'The health impacts of extractive industry transnational corporations: a study of Rio Tinto in Australia and Southern Africa', *Globalization and Health*, 15(13). Available at: https://doi.org/10.1186/s12992-019-0453-2

Anaf, J. *et al.* (2022) 'Assessing the health impacts of transnational corporations: a case study of Carlton and United Breweries in Australia', *Globalization and Health*, 18(80). Available at: https://doi.org/10.1186/s12992-022-00870-0

Anderson, T (2006) 'Policy coherence and conflict of interest: The OECD guidelines on health and poverty', *Critical Public Health*, 16(3), pp. 245–257. Available at: https://doi.org/10.1080/09581590600986473

Anderssen. E. (2010) 'The pink-ribbon backlash' *The Globe and Mail*, 17 October. Available at: www.theglobeandmail.com/life/health-and-fitness/the-pink-ribbon-backlash/articl e563272/ (Accessed: 10 February 2023).

Baum, F.E. *et al.* (2016) 'Assessing the health impact of transnational corporations: its importance and a framework' *Globalization and Health*, 12(27). Available at: https://doi.org/10.1186/s12992-016-0164-x

Bodini, C. *et al.* (2020) 'Methodological challenges in researching activism in action: civil society engagement towards health for all', *Critical Public Health*, 30(4), pp. 386–397. Available at: https://doi.org/10.1080/09581596.2019.1650892

Broom, A. *et al.* (2022) 'Antimicrobial resistance as a problem of values? Views from three continents', *Critical Public Health*, 31(4), pp. 451–463. Available at: https://doi.org/ 10.1080/09581596.2020.1725444

Broom, A. *et al.* (2023) 'Vulnerability and antimicrobial resistance', *Critical Public Health*, 33(3), pp. 308–317. Available at: https://doi.org/10.1080/09581596.2022.2123733

Buntz, B. (2021) 'Big Pharma resists international corporate tax proposal', *Pharmaceutical Processing World*, 27 July. Available at: www.pharmaceuticalprocessingworld.com/big-pharma-resists-international-corporate-tax-proposal/ (Accessed: 10 February 2023).

Campbell, C. and Cornish, F. (2021) 'Public health activism in changing times: re-locating collective agency', *Critical Public Health*, 31(2), pp. 125–133. Available at: https://doi.org/10.1080 /09581596.2021.1878110

Cohen, J. (1985) 'Strategy or identity: new theoretical paradigms and contemporary social movements', *Social Research*, 52(4), pp. 663–716.

Collier, R. (2010) 'Critics say UNCIEF-Cadbury partnership is mere sugarwashing', *Canadian Medical Association Journal*, 182(18), pp. E813–E814. Available at: https://doi.org/10.1503/cmaj.109-3720

Cornish, F. (2021) '"Grenfell changes everything?" Activism beyond hope and despair', *Critical Public Health*, 31(3), pp. 293–305. Available at: https://doi.org/10.1080/09581 596.2020.1869184

CSI Market (2023) 'Pfizer Inc's Annual Effective Tax Rate'. Available at: https://csimarket. com/stocks/singleProfitabilityRatiosy.php?code=PFE&itx (Accessed: 10 February 2023).

Erman, M. and Wingrove, P. (2023) 'Drug Companies face COVID cliff in 2023 as sales set to plummet', *Reuters*, 6 February. Available at:www.reuters.com/business/healthcare-pharmaceuticals/drug-companies-face-covid-cliff-2023-sales-set-plummet-2023-02-06/ (Accessed: 10 February 2023).

Fidler, D. (2007) 'A pathology of public health securitism: approaching pandemics as security threats', in A.F. Cooper, J.J. Kirton, and T. Schrecker (Eds.) *Governing global health: challenge, response, innovation*. Aldershot: Ashgate (Global Governance Series), pp. 41–66.

French M. *et al.* (2022) 'Corporate contact tracing as a pandemic response', *Critical Public Health*, 32(1), pp. 48–55. Available at: https://doi.org/10.1080/09581596.2020.1829549

Frenk J. and Moon S. (2013) 'Governance challenges in global health', *New England Journal of Medicine*, 368(10), pp. 936–942. Available at: https://doi.org/10.1056/NEJMra 1109339

Gagnon, M. and Labonté, R. (2011) 'Human rights in global health diplomacy: a critical assessment', *Journal of Human Rights*, 10(2), pp. 189–213. Available at: https://doi.org/ 10.1080/14754835.2011.569295

Global Justice Now (2018) '69 of the richest 100 entities on the planet are corporations, not governments, figures show'. Available at: www.globaljustice.org.uk/news/69-rich est-100-entities-planet-are-corporations-not-governments-figures-show/ (Accessed 10 February 2023).

Glover R.E. *et al.* (2022) 'How pharmaceutical and diagnostic stakeholders construct policy solutions to a public health "crisis": an analysis of submissions to a United Kingdom House of Commons inquiry into antimicrobial resistance', *Critical Public Health*, 33(2), pp. 197–206. Available at: https://doi.org/10.1080 /09581596.2022.2026296

Green, J. (2012) 'One health, one medicine' and critical public health', *Critical Public Health*, 22(4), pp. 377–381. Available at: Available at: https://doi.org/10.1080/09581 596.2012.723395

Green, J. (2019) 'Time to interrogate corporate interests in public health?', *Critical Public Health*, 29(3), pp. 257–259. Available at: https://doi.org/10.1080/09581596.2019.1587886

Gumbonzvanda, N., Gumbonzvanda, F. and Burgess, R.A. (2021) 'Decolonising the "safe space" as an African innovation: the Nhanga as quiet activism to improve women's health and wellbeing', *Critical Public Health*, 31(2), pp. 169–181. Available at: https://doi.org/10.1080/09581596.2020.1866169

Guo, C. *et al.* (2022) 'The effect of COVID-19 on public confidence in the World Health Organization: a natural experiment among 40 countries', *Globalization and Health* 18(77). Available at: https://doi.org/10.1186/s12992-022-00872-y

Hoffman S.J. *et al.* (2022) 'International treaties have mostly failed to produce their intended effects', *Proceedings of the National Academy of Sciences*, 119(32), p. e2122854119. Available at: https://doi.org/10.1073/pnas.2122854119

Horner, J., Wood, J.G. and Kelly, A. (2013) 'Public health in/as "national security": tuberculosis and the contemporary regime of border control in Australia', *Critical Public Health*, 23(4), pp. 418–431. Available at: https://doi.org/10.1080/09581596.2013.824068

Kajeepeta, S. *et al.* (2022) 'Policing the pandemic: estimating spatial and racialized inequities in New York City police enforcement of COVID-19 mandates', *Critical Public Health*, 32(1), pp. 56–67. Available at: https://doi.org/10.1080/09581596.2021.1987387

Kapilashrami, A. *et al.* (2022) 'Ethnic disparities in health and social care workers' exposure, protection, and clinical management of the COVID-19 pandemic in the UK', *Critical Public Health*, 32(1), pp. 68–81. Available at: https://doi.org/10.1080/09581596.2021.1959020

Kaul, I. (ed.) (2003) *Providing global public goods: managing globalization*. Oxford: Oxford University Press. Available at: https://doi.org/10.1093/0195157400.001.0001

Klein, N. (2007) *The shock doctrine: the rise of disaster capitalism*. Toronto: Knopf.

Labonté, R. (2008) 'Global health in public policy: finding the right frame?', *Critical Public Health*, 18(4), pp. 467–482. Available at: https://doi.org/10.1080/09581590802443588

Labonté, R. (2022) 'Ensuring global health equity in a post-pandemic economy', *International Journal of Health Policy and Management*, 11(8), pp. 1246–1250. Available at: https://doi.org/10.34172/ijhpm.2022.7212

Labonté, R. and Bodini, C. (eds.) (2022) *Global Health Watch 6: in the shadow of the pandemic*. London: Bloomsbury Press.

Labonté, R. and Laverack, G. (2008) *Health promotion in action: from local to global empowerment*. London: Palgrave Macmillan.

Labonté, R. and Ruckert, A. (2019) *Health equity in a globalizing era: past challenges, future prospects*. Oxford: Oxford University Press.

Lalani, H.S., Avorn, J. and Kesselheim, A.S. (2022) 'US taxpayers heavily funded the discovery of COVID-19 vaccines', *Clinical Pharmacology & Therapeutics*, 111(3), pp. 542–544. Available at: https://doi.org/10.1002/cpt.2344

Leach, M. *et al.* (2022) 'Rethinking disease preparedness: incertitude and the politics of knowledge', *Critical Public Health*, 32(1), pp. 82–96. Available at: https://doi.org/10.1080/09581596.2021.1885628

Lee, J. Kim, M-H. and Di Ruggiero, E. (2021) 'The corporate killing movement in South Korea: a critical realist analysis of social structure and collective agency', *Critical Public Health*, 31(2), pp. 156–168. Available at: https://doi.org/10.1080/09581596.2020.1838443

Lee, K. (2010) 'How do we move forward on the social determinants of health: the global governance challenges', *Critical Public Health*, 20(1), pp. 5–14. Available at: https://doi.org/10.1080 /09581590903563573

Macrotrends (2023) 'Pfizer Profit Margin 2020-2022'. Available at: www.macrotrends.net/stocks/charts/PFE/pfizer/profit-margins (Accessed: 10 February 2023).

Magnusson, R. and Patterson, D. (2021) 'Global action, but national results: strengthening pathways towards better health outcomes for non-communicable diseases', *Critical Public Health*, 31(4), pp. 464–476. Available at: https://doi.org/10.1080/09581596.2019.1693029

Marelli, L., Kieslich, K. and Geiger, S. (2022) 'COVID-19 and technosolutionism: responsibilization without contextualization?', *Critical Public Health*, 32(1), pp. 1–4. Available at: https://doi.org/10.1080 /09581596.2022.2029192

Moyo, D. (2009) *Dead Aid: why aid is not working and how there is a better way for Africa*. New York: Farrar, Straus and Giroux.

Mumford, E.L. *et al.* (2023) 'Evolution and expansion of the One Health approach to promote sustainable and resilient health and well-being: a call to action', *Frontiers in Public Health*, 10, pp. 1–13. Available at: https://doi.org/10.3389/fpubh.2022.1056459

Musoliro, C., Baum, F., Freeman, T., Labonté, R., Bodini, C. and Sanders, D. (2020) 'Global health activists' lessons on building social movements for Health for All', *International Journal for Health Equity*, 19(116), pp. 1–14. Available at: https://doi.org/10.1186 /s12959-020-01232-1

Mwacalimba, K.K. (2012) 'Globalised disease control and response distortion: a case study of avian influenza pandemic preparedness in Zambia', *Critical Public Health*, 22(4), pp. 391–405. Available at: https://doi.org/10.1080/09581596.2012.710739

Nature Microbiology (2020) 'Editorial: antimicrobial resistance in the age of COVID-19', *Nature Microbiology*, 5(779). Available at: https://doi.org/10.1038/s41564-020-0739-4

Offe, C. (1984) *Contradictions of the welfare state*. Boston: MIT Press.

Organization for Economic Cooperation and Development (OECD) (2003). *Poverty and health: DAC guidelines and reference series*. Paris: OECD (in association with the World Health Organization).

Ottersen, O.P. *et al.* (2014) 'The political origins of health inequity: prospects for change', *The Lancet*, 383(9917), pp. 630–667. Available at: https://doi.org/10.1016/S0140-6736(13)62407-1

Park, S.-J. *et al.* (2022) "Ebola is a business": an analysis of the atmosphere of mistrust in the tenth Ebola epidemic in the DRC', *Critical Public Health*, 33(3), pp. 297–307. Available at: https://doi.org/10.1080 /09581596.2022.2128990

Patnaik, P. (2023a) 'Choice facing countries: expand scope or preserve core functions? [Amendments to the International Health Regulations]', *Geneva Health Files: Newsletter Edition #15*. 21 February 2023. Available at: https://genevahealthfiles.substack.com/p/choice-facing-countries-expand-scope

Patnaik, P. (2023b) 'The zero draft of the pandemic accord: a discursive journey into equity', *Geneva Health Files: Newsletter Edition #14*. 8 February 2023. Available at: https://genevahealthfiles.substack.com/p/the-zero-draft-of-the-pandemic-accord

People's Working Group on Multistakeholderism (2022) 'The great takeover: a multisectoral mapping of multistakeholder institutions', 17 January. Available at: www.tni.org/en/publication/the-great-takeover

Pollock, A. (1995) 'Privatisation by stealth?', *Health Visitor*, 68(3), pp.98–99.

Powell, D. (2014) 'Childhood obesity, corporate philanthropy and the creeping privatisation of health education', *Critical Public Health*, 24(2), pp. 226–238. Available at: https://doi.org/10.1080 /09581596.2013.846465

Ribera-Almandoz, O. and Clua-Losada, M. (2021 'Health movements in the age of austerity: rescaling resistance in Spain and the United Kingdom', *Critical Public Health*, 31(2), pp. 182–192. Available at: https://doi.org/10.1080/09581596.2020.185 6333

Ruckert R. *et al.* (2016) 'Global health diplomacy: a critical review of the literature', *Social Science and Medicine*, 155, pp. 61–72. Available at: https://doi.org/10.1016/j.socscimed.2016.03.004.

Ruckert, A. *et al.* (2020) 'Governing antimicrobial resistance: a narrative review of global governance mechanisms', *Journal of Public Health Policy*, 41(4), pp. 515–528. Available at: https://doi.org/10.1057/s41271-020-00248-9

Sachs, J. (2014) 'The case for aid', *Foreign Policy*, 21 January. Available at: https://foreig npolicy.com/2014/01/21/the-case-for-aid/. (Accessed: 10 February 2023).

Sanders, D., Bodini, C. and Sengupta, A. (2019) *The contribution of civil society engagement to the achievement of health for all*. Available at: https://phmovement.org/wp-cont ent/uploads/2018/07/CSE4HFA_FinalReport_Short_180828.pdf

Sanders, D. *et al.* (2019) 'From primary health care to universal health coverage – one step forward and two steps back', *The Lancet*, 394, pp. 619–621. Available at: https://doi.org/ 10.1016 /S0140-6736(19)31831-8

Scambler, G and Kelleher, D. (2006) ['New social and health movements: issues of representation and change', *Critical Public Health*, 16(3), pp. 219–231. Available at: https://doi. org/10.1080 /09581590600986440

Speed, E., Carter, S. and Green, J. (2022) 'Pandemics, infection control and social justice: challenges for policy evaluation', *Critical Public Health*, 32(1), pp. 44–47. Available at: https://doi.org/10.1080 /09581596.2022.2029195

Tait, M. and Riediger, N. (2021) 'A sin tax on sugary drinks unfairly targets Indigenous communities instead of improving health', *The Conversation*, 21 February. Available at: https://theconversation.com/a-sin-tax-on-sugary-drinks-unfairly-targets-indigenous-communities-instead-of-improving-health-155108

The Lancet (2023) 'Editorial: One Health: a call for ecological equity', *The Lancet*, 401(10372), p. 169. Available at: https://doi.org/10.1016/S0140-6736(23)00090-9

Third World Network (2023) *WHO: Zero Draft of the pandemic instrument creates an "illusion" of equity*. Available at: www.twn.my/title2/health.info/2023/hi230207.htm

UNCTAD (2020) *Topsy-turvy world: net transfer of resources from poor to rich countries. Policy Brief No. 78*. Available at: https://unctad.org/publication/topsy-turvy-world-net-transfer-resources-poor-rich-countries

United Nations (2000). *United Nations Millennium Declaration*. New York: United Nations. Available at: www.ohchr.org/en/instruments-mechanisms/instruments/united-nations-mil lennium-declaration

Waugh, A. *et al.* (2022) 'How taxing sugary drinks reinforces weight stigma', *The Conversation*, 27 October. Available at: https://theconversation.com/how-taxing-sugary-drinks-reinforces-weight-stigma-192742

Wikipedia (no date) 'Companies committed to kids', *Wikipedia*. Available at: https:// en.wikipedia.org /wiki/Companies_Committed_to_Kids.

Wintrup, J. (2022) 'Outsourcing sovereignty: global health partnerships and the state in Zambia', *Critical Public Health*, 32(5), pp. 608–618. Available at: https://doi.org/ 10.1080/09581596.2021.1945535

World Health Organization (2015) *Global action plan on antimicrobial resistance*. Geneva: World Health Organization. Available at: https://iris.who.int/handle/10665/ 193736

World Health Organization (2023a) *WHO Framework Convention on Tobacco Control*. Available at: https://fctc.who.int/who-fctc/overview/parties (Accessed: 21 February 2023).

World Health Organization (2023b) *International Health Regulations*. Available at: www.who.int/health-topics/international-health-regulations#tab=tab_1 (Accessed: 21 February 2023).

Zak, D. (2021). '"Nothing ever ends": sorting through Rumsfeld's knowns and unknowns', *The Washington Post*, 1 July. www.washingtonpost.com/lifestyle/style/rumsfeld-dead-worcs-known-unknowns/2021/07/01/831175c2-d9df-11eb-bb9e-70fda8c37057_story.html

Zinsstag, J. *et al.* (2023), 'Advancing One human-animal-environment Health for global health security: what does the evidence say?' *The Lancet*, 401(10376), pp. 591–604. Available at: https://doi.org/10.1016/S0140-6736(22)01595-1

Zuboff, S. (2019). *The age of surveillance capitalism: the fight for a human future at the new frontier of power*. London: Profile Books.

8 Conclusion

We are all now (critical) political economists

Critical public health has always engaged with political economy in one way or another, whether focusing on the economic policies and practices that create the poverty or inequalities that underpin most diseases or the wealth/power drivers of gendered, racialized, and discriminating 'othering' that have long been commonplace and health hazardous. As the introduction and several chapters in this book discuss, there is a second and long-standing stream in critical public health scholarship that is more concerned with how knowledge is created and acted upon at the micro-level than with the political economy forces within which contingent health experiences arise. Given the 'turbulent times' that have accelerated since our original *Critical Perspectives in Public Health* book was published in 2008, this chapter focuses more on the importance of a political economy approach to understanding what remains critical to the public's health. We acknowledge, nonetheless, the necessity of a critical epistemology, one that allows for the productive deconstruction of hegemonic public health rooted in northern concerns and colonial relations (Breilh 2023). Indeed, as noted in the introduction chapter and in our final words below, the two stances complement one another and collectively underpin a robust field of critical public health scholarship.

Throughout this volume, the most commonly referenced political economy (a term used to describe where public policy and private economics meet) has been that associated with neoliberal capitalism. Globalization, as the previous two chapters recounted, was largely implemented as a neoliberal project. Liberal democracy, the dominant legitimating political paradigm in the west, was promoted (often imperiously) as the only viable model for a rules-based global international order. But, as Branko Milanovic, a Serbian-American economist with an astute sense of history, recently wrote (2025a):

> January 20, 2025, marks a symbolic end to global neoliberalism. Both of its components are gone. Globalism had now been converted into nationalism; neoliberalism has been made to apply to the economic sphere only ... Only low taxes, deregulation and worship of profit remain.

DOI: 10.4324/9781003654650-9

January 20, 2025, of course, was the day Donald Trump was sworn in for his second US presidency.

Trump's far-from-claimed landslide[1] came with a slim majority in both US legislative houses. For many, including those working in the public health sector, the election result was a shock. It was, however, confidently predictable to those following the rise of unfettered social media, the passive acceptance of lies as truth, and the huge explosion of techno-oligarch wealth, most of it tilted to Trump and the MAGA ('Make America Great Again') movement. More decisively, it was a result of the rise in inequalities, a decline in actual or perceived living standards and upward mobility, increased economic insecurity, and the four decades' failure of centrist and most centre-left (social democratic) parties to stand up to the immiserating impacts of globalization's neoliberal hegemony (The Guardian 2025; Piketty and Sandel 2025). What campaigning autocrats on the far right have done successfully is exaggerate the perceived losses of the traditional working class; merge it with masculinity's claimed 'woke' displacement by migrants, non-whites, and women; and mould it into wounded pride, humiliation, and anger (Haldar 2025).

The US is not alone in this drift to a far-right populism. Similar electoral shifts are taking place in the other epicentre of democratic (neo)-liberalism, the European Union, with similar overlays of misogyny, xenophobia, and white supremacy that characterizes the new Trump administration and much of its MAGA electoral base. At the time of writing (March 2025), ten European Union (EU) countries have hard-right and increasingly autocratic governments (Italy, Finland, Slovakia, Hungary, Croatia, Czech Republic, Belgium, Austria, Slovenia, and Turkey), with hard-right parties commanding large numbers of votes in several others, notably Germany (Coi 2024; Sevinc 2024). The 'cordon sanitaire' that EU centrist parties have used in the past to keep far-right parties out of power by refusing to rely upon their votes to govern is under increasing strain.

There is, as yet, no agreement on what the emergent system might be called that is being rushed into existence by Trump and the tech billionaires (the world's richest men) who are now running the world's most powerful nation.[2] But by the narrowest of margins, the US electorate in November 2024 voted in a misogynist, narcissistic, white supremacist bully keen only on his own self-interest and his exercise of imperial power. Liberal democracy chose a mean-spirited grifter with no regard for democratic norms or the rule of law and whose political agenda, apart from enriching himself and his tech 'broligarchs', as they have been called, is to eliminate any of the governmental checks (legal, administrative, regulatory, even constitutional) that might block his path to the dictatorship he has long hinted at wanting (Kirshner 2023). The combination of his funding cuts, deregulations, staff firings, ignored court rulings, and endless stream of executive orders centralizing power in his office, largely bypassing the two other branches of US government, is increasingly seen as a coup d'état. Democracy dies from within. The evisceration of an administrative state amidst demands for sworn loyalty from apparatchiks happened once before, in Germany in 1933. It did not end well then, and it is unlikely to do so now.

Neoliberal capitalism's toxic legacy

Although on a seeming ascendency, at some point in the not-so-distant future, Trump and other of the world's other autocrats will have to confront neoliberal capitalism's toxic legacy, even if their market fundamentalist policies in the near term will worsen it.[3] The term, polycrisis, described briefly in Chapter 7, first entered academic discourse in the 1990s, invoking complexity science and systems theory to argue that the many and worsening environmental, social, economic, and political crises threatening humankind were structurally interlinked (Tooze 2022). There is no shortage of crises that could be clustered under the single polycrisis neologism, which itself lacks meaningful definition (Lawrence et al. 2024). While some invoke the concept emphasizing the nature of a 'crisis' (a sudden event or series of events significantly harming the well-being of a large number of people) (Homer-Dixon et al. 2015), others criticize the term's popularized adoption for obscuring the role of capitalism and elite group interests in creating most of the collated crises (Sial 2023).

From that latter vantage, the past 40-plus years of neoliberal capitalism have accelerated at least three interrelated crises of ongoing public health import: increasing inequalities (income, wealth, resources), environmental collapse (climate chaos, biodiversity loss, species extinctions), and mass population movements (primarily with increasing numbers of people in the Global South seeking refuge from the first two). Elon Musk, Trump's apparent 'bagman', is poised to become the world's first trillionaire with others soon to follow, even as a billion people live with extreme hunger and near extreme poverty (Vargas 2024). Ecologically, in 2023 we crossed the 1.5-degree global warming 'red line' and are now transgressing six of the world's nine planetary life systems (Richardson et al. 2023), while the fossil fuel industries and their half-century of lying and dissembling (Center for Climate Integrity n.d.) with the collusion of enabling governments expand current production. The same year saw the number of people fleeing poverty, environmental catastrophe, violence, or all three rise to half a billion – the highest number ever recorded (Vince 2022). Many of these are internally displaced due to internationalized conflicts, a term for proxy wars between the world's multipolar powers, with the past five years each having the largest number of conflict-related deaths (excluding the 1994 Rwandan genocide) since the end of the Cold War (1989) (ACLED 2024).

The geopolitical context

The 'thirty golden years' following the end of the Second World War that began to wane in the 1970s before ending with the rise of neoliberalism in the 1980s, marked a taming of capitalist economics to that point. The US Roosevelt New Deal (1933–1938) enacted a series of domestic programmes, public works, and financial reforms and regulations to address the impacts of the Great Depression, post-war, which saw a dramatic compression in income inequalities in that country.

The New Deal is sometimes seen as similar in revolutionary scale and scope to its attempted terminal undoing by Trump's second presidency (Milanovic 2025b). Post-war parallel development in social democratic reforms took place in several European countries, heralding broader adoption across the developed economies of the global north of Keynesian economics and its emphasis on government management of markets, interventions to correct or prevent market failures, and economic stabilization via demand management and counter-cyclical public spending. Key features of this upending economic approach included high rates of progressive taxation and provision of state-funded public goods (health, education, housing, welfare) and strong regulatory oversight of the financial sector. These 'golden years', however, were also the dawn of the environmentally destructive and industrially polluting era of excess material consumption, a point to which this chapter returns (Labonté and Ruckert 2019), as well as the period of the Cold War (US/ Soviet Union), with both superpowers intervening militarily in many other countries, often inflicting gross health harms on people and planet. Their bipolar competition for standing as the global hegemon nonetheless gave rise to hybrid forms of state/market economic experiments in many of the decolonizing new nations, primarily in Africa in the 1960s.

This bipolar international order collapsed with the fall of the Berlin Wall in 1989, giving rise to a brief 'unipolar moment' dominated by the US and its projected 'liberal international order', i.e. neoliberalism. The unipolar moment faded quickly in the face of the 2008 global financial crisis and the COVID-19 pandemic in 2020, coupled with the economic rise of China over the same period, which has created the prevailing multipolar world (Ball 2019). If the EU is considered a single economic and political entity, most geopolitical scenarios describe an emerging global tri-polar order, with India potentially becoming a fourth regional anchor.

Despite its diminished geopolitical role, Russia continues to exert influence, indirectly through interference in other countries' elections (though it is not the only nation to do so), and more directly with its invasion of Ukraine, a response to the progressive eastward expansion of the North Atlantic Treaty Organization (NATO) deliberately seeking to isolate Russia. The Ukraine conflict is now widely seen as a proxy war between Russia and the liberal capitalist NATO nations led by the USA. Whether this proxy war, which can be seen as a new Cold War, becomes a 'hot war', or leads to some negotiated settlement, remains unknown, particularly given president-elect Trump's public displays of admiration for Russia's president Putin, willingness to surrender much of Russian-seized territory in Ukraine to Russia, and unwillingness to support Ukraine's NATO ambitions.

Also striking has been the economic rise of the BRICS countries (Brazil, Russia, India, China and South Africa), recently expanded to include Saudi Arabia, Qatar, Iran, Ethiopia, Indonesia, and Egypt to become BRICS+. Nearly 50 more countries indicate an interest to join. The current 11-nation club comprises 45% of the world's population and over 35% of global economic product (The Globalist 2024). It is attempting to de-dollarize its trade, especially amongst its members, emphasizing trade using its own currencies rather than the US dollar. It is also considering the creation of a BRICS+ currency similar to the euro, an unlikely outcome given member countries' varied economic and ideological commitments, but one that nonetheless has Trump threatening the group with '100 per cent tariffs' on all their exports if they do.

On the one hand, there is consensus that multilateralism is breaking down, abetted by the first Trump administration and rapidly worsening in the second Trump administration. The militarized chaos in the Middle East and the devastating loss of lives, livelihoods, and infrastructure, especially in Gaza, further impugn the ineffectiveness of our present multilateral governance systems (such as the UN Security Council). On the other hand, this new global multipolarity and rearranging of country alignments may lead to new efforts by the world's largest and middle-power states to reach some agreement on health governance in a new global order. One thing is certain: the 'American Century' is over, and the USA, despite its still overwhelming military strength, is no longer the global hegemon. Whether the second Trump administration, with its imperialist intents (Greenland, Canada, Panama Canal, Gaza), is attempting to regain that unipolar status or will accept a multipolar and globally anarchic world order, or one in which the US reclaims 'manifest destiny' over the entire Americas and leaves the rest of the world to be carved up into competing spheres of influence by other great powers, is yet to be known.

The alt-right war on health

As the geopolitical opera unfolds, and using Trump 2.0 and his flurry of executive orders as a proxy for the socio-economic and political agenda of much (if not most) of the new alt-right, it is quickly apparent the health threat posed by this agenda: withdrawal from the World Health Organization (WHO), the International Health Regulations, and the Pandemic Accord. Key US firings monitoring of the spread of H5N1 avian influenza across the USA and non-participation in global monitoring efforts places not only US citizens at risk, but much of the rest of the world should H5N1 become pandemic. The appointment of a conspiracy theorist and vaccine sceptic (Robert F Kennedy Jr) as health secretary (Wilkinson and Fairchild 2016)[4], the suspension of active health research grants, and other cuts to the National Institutes of Health compound these risks. US withdrawal from the WHO could lead other member states to do likewise; Argentina has already stated its intent to do so. More immediately, as the US is the single largest funder of WHO, many of the organization's programmes are in immediate jeopardy.

Dismantling of sexual and reproductive health rights (SRHR), such as Trump's reinstatement of the Global Gag Rule which bars US foreign assistance to organizations that provide, support, or even discuss abortion services, is another blow to global health. This decision severely limits women's access to essential health care, leading to increased maternal mortality, higher rates of unplanned pregnancies, and a rise in unsafe abortions. Since other countries oppose SRHR on similar, if different, religious rationales than those invoked by Trump and his evangelical Christian base, one can expect further erosion globally in existing SRHR implementation.

Trump's attacks on SRHR coincide with (temporary) freezing, drastic cuts to, and potential elimination of foreign aid. Although often used as an extension of US imperialism, the sudden freezing of funds will worsen humanitarian crises with catastrophic long-term consequences and has already led to a lack of antiretroviral (ARVs) in much of Africa (the USA has been the largest funder of HIV/AIDS programmes in much of the developing world, allowing it to exert significant 'soft power'). Feminists and critical health activists have long warned of the dangers of the anti-SRHR agenda, which is not just about health care but part of a broader effort to control women, LGBTQI+ individuals, and other marginalized populations. Trans people, women, refugees, and migrants are seen as threats to a stoked resurgence in 'masculinity'.

The USA is not alone in cutting foreign aid (technically referred to as Official Development Assistance, or ODA), a trend that accelerated post-pandemic. The UK in 2013, one of the few donor countries to reach the foreign aid target of 0.7% of gross domestic product (GDP), will cut its spending by 40% to just 0.3% of GDP in order to increase defence spending. This is widely seen as an attempt to appease Trump (Sabbagh 2025). Several other European donor nations have also cut their aid disbursements, including the Nordic countries (long the most proportionately generous), Germany, France, and the EU itself (Gulrajani and Pudussery 2025). ODA is not a panacea for the global maldistribution of wealth, the legacy of colonial exploitation, and continuing economic colonialization, and too often, it has served more as influential 'soft power' or subsidies to donor countries' domestic 'aid industry'. In that sense, the collapse in US foreign aid will force many US aid-dependent countries to diversify their pool of external financial contributions and their public resource allocations to meet their national health needs (Montenegro and Fonseca 2025). But the rapid decrease in levels of aid translates directly to increased health risks, disproportionately impacting women and girls in aid-recipient countries (Lay 2025), with spillover impacts on many other countries.

Within hours of reclaiming the presidency, Trump withdrew the USA from the 2015 Paris Agreement on climate change, terminated funding for developing countries to mitigate climate impacts, and is fast-tracking fossil fuel projects. His multimillionaire energy secretary heads up a fossil fuel company and claims that 'there is no climate crisis' and that 'net zero' emission targets are 'sinister'. The hugely inequitable health impacts of this last gasp embrace of a deadly addiction to hydrocarbon energy are well known, as is the pace of its worsening and its pushing of eight billion people out of the habitable climate niche with each one-degree temperature rise. Trump's climate policies are a more extreme rerun of his first presidency (Anderson 2025). Though no other countries withdrew from the Paris Agreement or their commitments then, there is concern that they may begin to do so now. Many of the corporate and financial sectors' 'net zero' pledges have already been scaled back or withdrawn, with several of the world's largest fossil fuel companies (such as BP) slashing their green energy investments and pivoting back to oil and gas with new multi-billion dollar investments (Ambrose 2025). The energy transition, while slowed down, is not thought to be in terminal peril

(Bremmer 2025), although whether it can survive Trump's presidency (or dictatorship) before irremediable climate collapse is a deeply troubling unknown.

Trump has declared trade war on most of the USA's trading partners, proposing massive tariffs often with no apparent trade-relevant reason. Canada's threatened tariffs are putatively for allowing fentanyl and illegal migrants to cross its shared border with the USA, a claim for which there is no factual basis. Although China (now the main economic and geopolitical competitor to the USA) is the main target, there is irony in that it was Republican and other neocon leaders' promotion of globalized neoliberalism that led US (and European) manufacturing to outsource to China in the first place, creating the capital and technological transfer that allowed it to become the second most powerful country in the world. Trump's neomercantilist tariffs will hurt other countries (especially when companies re-shore to the USA to avoid tariff-related profit losses) but will also hurt American consumers. While heterodox economists have long forewarned of the economic devastation of a second Trump presidency, some neoliberal economists are now modelling how the proposed tariffs alone will reduce US and global economic growth (not necessarily a bad thing, as will be discussed later) and lead to even higher US trade deficits (Trump's argued trade reason for imposing tariffs) (Lachman 2025). Trade wars in the past have become world wars, and therein lies the more existential, longer-term health threat.

The negative impacts of tariffs will be amplified by Trump's commitment to further and deeper corporate tax cuts, which will increase health-harming inequality and poverty. Indeed, apart from tariffs being part of Trump's imperialist threats to other nations, they are intended to offset his tax cuts that will disproportionately and hugely benefit the wealthiest Americans and corporations (Clausing 2025). It will also fuel inflation not only in the USA, but internationally. The 'Department of Government Efficiency' (DOGE) (a more radical cost-cutting version of neoliberal austerity), the Trump/Musk drive to deregulate, and the promised tax cuts (up to a mooted elimination of all taxation) have been picked up by corporations and alt-right parties demanding the same in other countries. In addition to austerity around public services and supports, tax cuts usually lead to more public borrowing, which directly or indirectly increases the profitability of lending or investing banks and private equity funds and further widens the socially destabilizing gap between the fractional 1 per cent and the rest.

Amidst this chaos lies a larger opportunity presented by the sheer scale of Trump's Agenda 2025 disruptions to and dissolution of the post-war global economic order. The resulting economic, political, and social chaos and turbulence create space for advancing different ideas of how political economies might be structured, a point we return to shortly.

The attack on truth

Critical public health, as many of this book's chapters discuss, is agnostic on the concept of 'truth', arguing how our understanding of reality is socially constructed and filtered through many screens, although for most critical scholars that there is a reality, even if not definitively knowable, is not in question. What the second Trump presidency is unleashing is an attack on 'truth' far more violent and extensive than the past decade's right-wing 'anti-woke' purge of culturally liberal and socially just ideas and the political reforms and activist movements that supported them. The male backlash and its misogynist and 'othering' roots were gifted a huge boost with Trump's rapid elimination of all US government agencies' DEI (diversity, equity and inclusion) initiatives, a move emulated by the tech social media giants and American corporations. The Department of Education, headed now by the former CEO of the World Wrestling Federation, is being told to ensure that anything remotely promoting DEI values needs to be stripped from school and university curricula, or they lose federal funding (Associated Press 2025). Lists of books to be banned from public libraries are being created. The anti-DEI momentum reached a nadir when the US Secretary of State boycotted the G20 summit in South Africa, complaining that the G20 was promoting "very bad things ... solidarity, equality and sustainability" (RCI 2025).

The breadth of this attack is numbing. US government websites have been removed or stripped of any content remotely concerned with issues of climate or justice: government employees (at least those not yet fired or compelled to resign) are forbidden or fearful to speak out of Musk's DOGE destruction of the bureaucratic administrative state; research grants are frozen, data stripped from public sites, and scientists muzzled in their ability to report findings not approved by Trump s appointed overseers. Fact-checking has been eliminated on social media sites owned by the tech 'broligarchs' that funded and continue to financially support Trump's presidency in anticipation of a surge in already obscene profits with promised tax cuts and deregulation. Amazon billionaire Jeff Bezos, owner of the Washington Post, is restricting the paper's opinion section's articles only to those "in support and defence of ... personal liberties and free markets", shuttering any critical analysis of the Trump agenda. The Post's opinion editor resigned in protest

For public health researchers and activists, one disturbing aspect of Trump's 2025 ideological remaking of the world is its retreat from rationality, science, and evidence. University academics, considered by definition to be elitist 'woke' Marxist DEI radicals, are being silenced or pre-emptively shuttering themselves. We find ourselves confronted by a new era of 'the big lie', where whatever 'big enough'[5] belligerent and demonstrable falsehoods are repeatedly uttered by Trump, or his appointees, are amplified through right-wing mainstream and social media as 'truths', while statements fact-checked with evidence are rebutted as 'lies'. George Orwell is once more vindicated.

There is considerable grit in all the above for critical public health researchers, scholars, and activists to continue working on. For one, there is historical, hypothetical, and opinion survey evidence suggesting that steep inequalities and stoking of emotive (and not rational) forces are what led to Trump's second election and that of his autocratic fellow travellers. But there is little (at least recent) in-depth study of how these intersecting vectors of insecurity, 'othering', and a manipulated victimhood explain why so many choose abhorrent 'big men'. It is also probable that the individual 'responsibilization' for health that other chapters have linked to neoliberalism will be retained in whatever the new alt-right political order becomes. The imminent demise of international trade law (or at least prior norms) presents some opportunities for critical health engagement with new trade norms and rules, opposing those that differentially benefit the already wealthy and powerful and realigning trade routes that support the eco-just aims gaining popular support globally.

Emphatically, this is not a time for those of us with the capacity to rabble-rouse to keep one's head low, hoping to wait it out. Rather, as increasing numbers of academics, government workers, civil society organization members are doing, speaking out, protesting, and taking some form of direct action are now some of the most 'critical' of public health practices we need to embrace. As one of us recently wrote, public health can no longer fence-sit politically (Labonté 2024a).

The rise and fall of neoliberalism: Is an emancipatory well-being economy possible?

As noted earlier in this chapter, there is as yet no consensus on what economic system Trump's (and his fellow autocrats') upheaval of the 20th-century international liberal order might be. Capitalism, however, in the short term, will still dominate national, if not also international, economies. Oligarchic capitalism? Neomercantilist capitalism? Authoritarian state capitalism? Mafia capitalism? There are certainly elements of all of this, as well as of rentier capitalism (the oligarchic model) or what Varoufakis calls technofeudalism (where the tech and soon-to-be AI rentiers essentially control access rights to most of the world's resources, bringing any semblance of market capitalism to a close) (Varoufakis 2024). It is unlikely but not impossible to see a return of 'Zombie Neo-liberalism' much as what happened after neoliberalism's presumed defeat following the 2008 financial crisis and recession failed to stick (Wolf 2023), at least until Trump's first electoral win.

It is equally unlikely to return to a neo-Keynesian democratic capitalism even if it becomes plastered with the vast number of ameliorating reforms that might keep civil society in affluent nations minimally content and the worst rapaciousness of short-term capital extractivism sufficiently checked to prevent a climate and economic breakdown of such force that it precipitates a civilizational collapse (Kirshner 2023). This implies that many of the initial economic reform mantras that followed the COVID-19 pandemic, which could have ushered in Keynesian 2.0 with their promise to 'build back better', are ultimately inadequate in the analytical eyes of many CPH researchers; they are also now confronting an alt-right headwind of unexpected fury.

As Trump's staged turmoil is still unfolding, it is hard to know how much of it will eventually survive US court challenges or international vituperation. But Gramsci's oft-misquoted comment on the *zeitgeist* of the 1930s – that 'the old world is dying and the new world struggles to be born ... now is the time of monsters'[6] – captures a sentiment shared by many in public health. What 'new world' might health activists embrace and advocate for in this time of posturing monsters?

A number of candidates have been proposed, albeit before Trump's affirmed second presidency, two of which have received considerable attention and both of which assume a reformed capitalism of differing degrees of radicalism. Mazzucato's promotion of 'mission economies' calls for strong, participatory governments to actively shape markets to achieve socially desirable outcomes (e.g. in climate, health, prosperity) (Mazzucato 2021) rather than simply respond to capitalism's inevitable market failures. The Club of Rome's collaborative 2022 *Earth4All Report* (Club of Rome 2023) returns to its classic 1972 report, *The Limits to Growth* (Meadows et al. 1972) the first attempt to model the environmental outcomes of a consumption trajectory at the scale unleashed by advances in industrial technologies in the 1950s. The 2022 Report repeats and updates the earlier report's 1972 econometric modelling, projecting two different scenarios. The first it calls 'too little too late' which assumes a continued tinkering with the margins of consumptogenic capitalism that eventually leads us to civilizational collapse; and a second labelled the 'great leap' option that foresees acceptance of a spate of tax, regulatory, and public good measures leaving us in 2100 with a healthy and still human-liveable planet. That science and ethics underpin both candidates renders them anathema to the alt-right, at least for the near term, but they are sufficiently hopeful to ignore, albeit with critique, and to internalize as viable options to the monsters of the moment.

Both candidates reference degrowth (or what others have called postgrowth), a concept first coined in the 1970s that entered more common economic discourse post-2008. Rejected by classical economists for whom growth (green or otherwise) is the essence of any economy (capitalist or otherwise), degrowth challenges the ethical and empirical viability of the post-war's '30 golden years' of rapidly escalating and economically inequitable consumption of finite planetary resources. It seeks to overturn the hegemony of conventional growth through a democratically led redistributive downscaling of production and consumption and an equitable reallocation of wealth, both within and across countries and between present and future generations. It is not anti-growth per se, but opposes growth in consumption of material resources that are unnecessary for human well-being and that risk irreversible ecosystem damage. Many of the economic activities that drive current conventional measures of growth would have to be abandoned (i.e. regulated downwards to rapid non-existence), while other growth-related activities (e.g. greening our energy systems, actively revitalizing damaged ecosystems, embracing the low-consumption and historically undervalued caring economy) would thrive.

There is some concern that the negative connotation of 'degrowth' works poorly as a mobilizing strategy (Meurs et al. 2023) and that alternatives for marketing the concept could include 'fair growth' or 'regenerative good growth' (Pretty et al. 2025) for their more positive affirmation of prosperity and abundance. In parallel with efforts to describe an eco-just and health-promoting political economy, another term has entered public health discourse: the 'well-being economy' (Labonté 2024b). In simplest terms, a well-being economy is one that pursues an equitable global allocation of the resources people need for a healthy life while staying within the ecological limits of our planet.

The *Earth4All* collaboration describes its policy agenda as a well-being economy, as does the WHO's Council on the Economics of Health for All (2020–2022), comprised of some of the world's most outspoken heterodox and feminist economists. The Council's various reports provide an evidence-informed list of recommendations that would be familiar to many critical public health scholars and advocates, who have long argued for tax and environmental justice, economic fairness, gender equity, collective human rights, food security, and properly financed governments protecting and expanding the space for public engagement in policymaking. The intent of the Council's work is to "transform economic systems and co-create an economic policy design guide to shift societal success beyond GDP growth and instead deliver shared wellbeing" (WHO Council on the Economics of Health for All 2023, p. 24).

Well-being itself is hardly a new idea, in Western societies dating at least to the writings of ancient Greek philosophers. It is also found in expressions in many different cultures and figures in the founding Constitution of the WHO (1948) and its classic definition of health "as state of complete physical, social and mental well-being, and not merely the absence of disease or infirmity" (p. 1). Well-being, in turn, at least in WHO parlance, "encompasses quality of life, as well as the ability of people and societies to contribute to the world in accordance with a sense of meaning and purpose" (WHO 2021, p. 10). Setting aside that there are numerous ways in which well-being might be and has been characterized, it is generally accepted to be a positive and desired state.

The idea of a well-being economy, however, is new and binds the experience of well-being (however it might be defined) to the economic policies that support it, particularly "the equitable distribution of resources" that allow for "overall thriving, and [environmental] sustainability" (WHO 2021, p. 10). As with the degrowth concept, there is some international momentum behind these ideas, including the 2018 founding of a Wellbeing Economy Alliance with over 200 member organizations. Amongst these members is a small group of countries whose governments formed a network of Wellbeing Economy Governments (WEGo) (Finland, Scotland, Wales, Iceland, and New Zealand). As well, since 2021 the Euro WHO office has supported the development of policy-level understanding of well-being economies across the EU region, alongside other WEGo countries (Labonté 2024b). By one estimate, a majority of governments of the Organization for Economic Cooperation and Development (OECD) (the club of rich nations) are engaged in developing or using some form of well-being measures within their policymaking, albeit with the risk of performative change only in which a well-being economy becomes a matter of reporting on a new set of indicators with little attention to enacting the changes in policies or economic practices implied by such measures. At present, the alt-right upending of the liberal economic order might well dampen even these slender initiatives.

At the same time, however, capitalism's toxic polycrisis might also see a resurgent left populism push politics in a different direction, one in which the well-being economy's " 'positive language' of abundance, wellness, and conviviality, with a view to building a forward-looking narrative of opportunities for human creativity, thus inspiring collective action and making governments more amenable to policy change" (Costanza 2020). As Labonté (2024b) has written:

> With a strong emphasis on living in harmony with nature a well-being economy has global resonance, from the Latin-American *buen vivir* to the South African *ubuntu*, the Swedish *lagom*, and values associated with Buddhism and Confucianism. It is also very consonant with the (critical) public health literature on social determinants of health, and the long-standing community empowerment tenets of many health promotion and social welfare programs and practices. In that sense, the current promotion of well-being economics is something both ancient (and hence renewed) but also new (embedding within it an implicit or occasionally explicit critique of status quo economics, with an emphasis on collective and not just individual well-being).
>
> (p. 5)

Are states likely to embrace the challenge a well-being economy presents to capitalism's consumptogenic and predatory practices? Marxist health political economists largely answer in the negative. There is too much historical evidence of states colluding with, rather than forcibly challenging, the short-term interests of capital apart from tossing a few mildly redistributive policy crumbs in the direction of the marginalized (Waitzkin 2023). The modern state that arose following the 1648 Treaty of Westphalia that ended Europe's religious wars emerged at the same time as capitalism; state and market have been conjoined ever since.

In contrast to reform-oriented stances associated with some of the structural theorizing of a well-being economy, where some form of capitalism is accepted as a base from which to build, more radical models have been well-defined. One of these is ecosocialism, in which the tenets of socialist economics entwine with the agroecological feminism found in many Indigenous knowledge systems. Ecosocialism has been advanced as a more trenchant base from which actions should arise. Löwy (2018) notes:

> In synthesizing the basic tenets of ecology and the Marxist critique of political economy, ecosocialism offers a radical alternative to an unsustainable status quo. Rejecting a capitalist definition of "progress" based on market growth and quantitative expansion ... it advocates policies founded on non-monetary criteria, such as social needs, individual well-being, and ecological equilibrium.
>
> (p. 1)

Many ecosocialist movements argue the importance of prefigurative action, combining a loud and continuous discrediting critique of the prevailing capitalist with immediate 'doable' creation of and support for localized forms of non-commodified (non-capitalist) economic systems (e.g. local or non-currency systems of exchange, various forms of cooperatives, environmental sustainability projects). As Breilh (2023) puts it, what is needed is a "real project of justice and the full ethics of life"

(p. 16) rooted in critique of both the global economy and the bioethics of conventional public health. Such initiatives 'prefigure' what a transformed economic system might look like, if achieved by revolution, evolution, or ecological necessity at political scale. It is precisely at this intersection of macro and micro that the two streams in critical public health converge. Building a nuanced understanding of how powerful knowledge and social collective systems arise in contingent local contexts is important for advancing prefigurative actions, while a continuing exposition of the barriers and opportunities for healthful change that might exist within our fracturing political economy structures defines well the 21st agenda for critical public health. It also names the self-care tonic needed to avoid Gramsci's 'pessimism of the intellect' overwhelming the 'optimism of the will'.

Notes

1 Of votes cast for president, Trump received 49.8%, Harris 48.3%. But only 63.9% of eligible voters voted, meaning Trump's share of eligible voters is less than 32% (Lindsay 2024).
2 In the first month following the Trump election, Elon Musk's wealth grew by $170 billion, to $455 billion (Marcus 2024).
3 Not all autocrats fit neatly into the alt-right frame. Some emerge from progressive populist uprisings initially claiming more alt-left and communalist ideologies before leaders adopt a 'strong man' authoritarianism. Nicaragua's Ortega and Venezuela's Maduro come to recent mind.
4 Conspiracy theories can sometimes convey 'truths' or have meaning about other things, leading to different patterns of and rationales for resistance to public health measures, as described in a study of resistance to Ebola responses in two West African countries (Wilkinson and Fairhead 2016). Since the COVID-19 pandemic, however, vaccine scepticism has been embedded in far-right extremist politics. In Kennedy's appointment, there is an opportunity for critical engagement with the 'how' and 'why' of anti-traditional public health framings of disease cause and health risk. Kennedy's 'make America healthy' again campaign also expresses concern with the health consequences of ultra-processed foods which, if directed to regulating corporate control over food production, could constitute a public health 'win'. But within the Trump administration's deregulation agenda and given its alignment with the US transnational corporations that dominate global good production, Kennedy's concern with unhealthy goods is more likely to manifest as the individual responsibilization discussed in Chapter 3.
5 The political strategy of the big lie is often attributed to Nazi propagandist, Joseph Goebbels, who is reputed to have written that

> If you tell a lie big enough and keep repeating it, people will eventually come to believe it. The lie can be maintained only for such time as the State can shield the people from the political, economic and/or military consequences of the lie. It thus becomes vitally important for the State to use all of its powers to repress dissent, for the truth is the mortal enemy of the lie, and thus by extension, the truth is the greatest enemy of the State.

There is no evidence he actually said this, but little doubting that the technique it captures was utilized by Hitler and the Nazis and by autocrats both before and after. In Trump's first presidency, when his aides questioned the false statements that he ordered them to

broadcast and repeat, he would reply: " ... as long as you keep repeating something, it doesn't matter what you say" (Baker 2025). Hannah Arendt, one of the most influential political theorists of the 20th century who wrote evocatively of the 'banality of evil' with reference to the Nazis, in her last public interview noted that the power of the big lie 'is not that you believe the lies, but rather that nobody believes anything anymore' which is what 'makes it possible for a totalitarian or any other dictatorship to rule' (Berkowitz 2024).
6 The actual passage from Gramsci's prison notebooks reads, 'The old is dying and the new cannot be born: in this interregnum the most varied morbid phenomena occur'.

References

ACLED (2024) *Global conflicts double over the past five years*. Armed Conflict Location & Event Data. Available at: https://acleddata.com/conflict-index/

Ambrose, J. (2025) 'BP blames "misplaced" faith in green transition for its renewed focus on fossil fuels', *The Guardian*, 26 February. Available at: www.theguardian.com/business/2025/feb/26/bp-oil-and-gas-spending-green-energy-scale-back

Anderson, S. (2025) 'The US exits the climate fight – can others fill the vacuum?', *Health Policy Watch*, 22 January. Available at: https://healthpolicy-watch.news/the-united-states-exits-the-climate-fight/

Associated Press (2025) 'Trump administration gives schools deadline to cut DEI or lose federal funds', *The Guardian*, 18 February. Available at: www.theguardian.com/us-news/2025/feb/18/trump-administration-schools-dei-programs-deadline

Baker, P. (2025) 'In Trumps alternate reality, lies and distortion drive change' *New York Times*, February 25. Available at: www.nytimes.com/2025/02/23/us/politics/trump-alternative-reality.html

Ball, J. (2019) '12 predictions for global geopolitics for 2019 through 2025—and beyond', *Global Security Review*. Available at: https://globalsecurityreview.com/world-will-look-like-2025/

Berkowitz, R. (2024) 'On fake Hannah Arendt quotations' *Amor Mundi – Hannah Arendt Center for Politics and Humanities*. Available at: https://hac.bard.edu/amor-mundi/on-fake-hannah-arendt-quotations-2024-08-04

Breilh, J. (2023) 'The social determination of health and the transformation of rights and ethics: A meta-critical methodology for responsible and reparative science', *Global Public Health*, 18(1), p. 2193830. Available at: https://doi.org/10.1080/17441692.2023.2193830

Bremmer, I. (2025) 'Trump will not kill the global energy transition', *Project Syndicate*, 11 February. Available at: www.project-syndicate.org/commentary/trump-will-not-kill-global-energy-transition-by-ian-bremmer-2025-02

Center for Climate Integrity (n.d.) 'Deception Documents'. Center for Climate Integrity (online). Available at: https://climateintegrity.org/deception-documents.

Clausing, K. (2025) 'The real reason President Trump pushes tariffs', *The New York Times*, 21 February. Available at: www.nytimes.com/2025/02/21/opinion/trump-tariffs-tax-cuts.html

Club of Rome (2023) Earth4All Report: September 2022-September 2023. Available at: https://earth4all.life /wp-content/uploads/2023/10/Earth4All_Activity_Report_2023.pdf

Coi, G. (2024) 'Mapped: Europe's rapidly rising right', *Politico*, 24 May. Available at: www.politico.eu/article/mapped-europe-far-right-government-power-politics-eu-italy-finalnd-hungary- parties-elections-polling/

Costanza, R. (2020) 'Ecological economics in 2049: getting beyond the argument culture to the world we all want', *Ecological Economics*, 168, p. 106484. Available at: https://doi.org/10.1016/j.ecolecon.2019.106484

Gulrajani, N. and Pudussery, J. (2025) 'With the knives out on development spending, have we reached "peak aid"?', *The Guardian*, 23 January. Available at: www.theguardian.com/global-development/2025/jan/23/global-development-economics-donor-spending-refugee-oecd-world-bank-peak-aid

Haldar, A. (2025) 'What is MAGAnomics?', *Project Syndicate*, 10 February. Available at: www.project-syndicate.org/commentary/maganomics-intellectual-grab-bag-for-political-messaging-not-economic-results-by-antara-haldar-2025-02

Homer-Dixon, T. *et al.* (2015) 'Synchronous failure: the emerging causal architecture of global crisis', *Ecology and Society*, 20(3), p. art6. Available at: https://doi.org/10.5751/ES-07681-200306

Kirshner, J. (2023) 'Rigged capitalism and the rise of pluto-populism: on Martin Wolf's "The Crisis of Democratic Capitalism"', *Los Angeles Review of Books*, 14 May. Available at: https://lareviewofbooks.org /article/rigged-capitalism-and-the-rise-of-pluto-populism-on-martin-wolfs-the-crisis-of-democratic- capitalism/

Labonté, R. (2024a) 'Public health can no longer fence-sit politically', *Canadian Journal of Public Health*, 115(5), pp. 701–704. Available at: https://doi.org/10.17269/s41997-024-00941-2

Labonté, R. (2024b) 'Can a well-being economy save us?', *International Journal of Health Policy and Management*, 13(1), pp. 1–6. Available at: https://doi.org/10.34172/ijhpm.8507.

Labonté, R. and Ruckert, A. (2019) *Health equity in a globalizing era: past challenges, future prospects*. First edition. Oxford New York: Oxford University Press.

Lachman, D. (2025) 'Trump's looming deficit disaster', *Project Syndicate*, 11 February. Available at: www.project-syndicate.org/commentary/trump-economic-policies-will-increase-us-trade-and-budget-deficits-by-desmond-lachman-2025-02

Lawrence, M. *et al.* (2024) 'Global polycrisis: the causal mechanisms of crisis entanglement', *Global Sustainability*, 7, p. e6. Available at: https://doi.org/10.1017/sus.2024.1

Lay, K. (2025) 'Starmer's cuts to UK aid budget are "cruel and shameful", say experts', *The Guardian*, 25 February. Available at: www.theguardian.com/global-development/2025/feb/25/starmer-cuts-to-uk-aid-budget-defence-trump-cruel-and-shameful-say-experts

Lindsay, J. (2024) The 2024 Election by the Numbers. Council on Foreign Relations. Available at: www.cfr.org/article/2024-election-numbers

Löwy, M. (2018) *Why ecosocialism: for a red-green future*. Great Transition Initiative. Available at: www.greattransition.org/images/Lowy-Why-Ecosocialism.pdf

Marcus, J. (2024) 'Elon Musk's wealth jumps by $170bn since election after he backed Trump with $277m', *The Independent*, 16 December. Available at: www.independent.co.uk/news/world/americas/elon-musk-net-worth-trump-b2665395.html

Mazzucato, M. (2021) *Mission economy: a moonshot guide to changing capitalism*. London: Allen Lane, an imprint of Penguin Books.

Meadows, D. *et al.* (1972) *The limits to growth: a report for the club of Rome's project on the predicament of mankind*. Hanover, Dartmouth College: Club of Rome.

Meurs, M., Koutsoumpa, M. and Huisman, V. (2023) 'Ensuring global health equity in a post-pandemic economy: words count! comment on "ensuring global health equity in a post-pandemic economy"', *International Journal of Health Policy and Management*, 12, p. 7794. Available at: https://doi.org/10.34172 /ijhpm.2023.7794

Milanovic, B. (2025a) ' "To the Finland Station" ', *Substack – Global Inequality and More 3.0*, 6 January. Available at: https://branko2f7.substack.com/p/to-the-finland-station?utm_source=substack& utm_medium=email

Milanovic, B. (2025b) 'Trump, the state and the revolution', *Substack – Global Inequality and More 3.0*, 15 February. Available at: https://branko2f7.substack.com/p/trump-the-state-and-the-revolution

Montenegro, C. and Fonseca, S. (2025) ' "Stop looking north, look to the world". Can we imagine Global Health without the USA at its centre?', *PLOS – Speaking of Medicine and Health*, 14 February. Available at: https://speakingofmedicine.plos.org/2025/02/14/stop-looking-north-look-to-the-world-can-we-imagine-global-health-without-the-usa-at-its-centre/

Piketty, T. and Sandel, M.J. (2025) *Equality: what it means and why it matters*. Cambridge: Polity.

Pretty, J. *et al.* (2025) 'How the concept of "regenerative good growth" could help increase public and policy engagement and speed transitions to net zero and nature recovery', *Sustainability*, 17(3), p. 849. Available at: https://doi.org/10.3390/su17030849

RCI (2025) 'U.S. to boycott next G20 meeting in South Africa', *Radio-Canada International – CBC News*, 7 February. Available at: https://ici.radio-canada.ca/rci/en/news/2138572/u-s-to-boycott-next-g20-meeting-in-south-africa

Richardson, K. *et al.* (2023) 'Earth beyond six of nine planetary boundaries', *Science Advances*, 9(37), p. eadh2458. Available at: https://doi.org/10.1126/sciadv.adh2458

Sabbagh, D. (2025) 'Starmer can only hope slashing aid to boost defence wins Trump's favour', *The Guardian*, 25 February. Available at: www.theguardian.com/politics/2025/feb/25/starmer-can-only-hope-aid-grab-raid-to-lift-defence-budget-wins-trumps-favour

Sevinc, N.T. (2024) '2025: Will the far right break through Europe's "cordon sanitaire"?', *Anadolu Ajansı (AA)*, 30 December. Available at: www.aa.com.tr/en/europe/2025-will-the-far-right-break-through-europe-s-cordon-sanitaire-/3438061

Sial, F. (2023) 'Whose polycrisis?', *Developing Economics*, 27 January. Available at: https://developingeconomics.org/2023/01/27/whose-polycrisis/

The Globalist (2024) 'BRICS Vs. the G7', *The Globalist*, 23 October. Available at: www.theglobalist.com/brics-brics-g7-economy-population-just-the-facts/#:~:text=BRICS%20member%20states%20now%20represent,)%20only%20account%20for%2010%25.&text=The%20BRICS%20countries%20account%20for,the%20G7%20only%20represents%2030%25

The Guardian (2025) 'The Guardian view on globalisation and its discontents: how the left was left behind', *The Guardian*, 13 January. Available at: www.theguardian.com/commentisfree/2025/jan/13/the-guardian-view-on-globalisation-and-its-discontents-how-the-left-was-left-behind

Tooze, A. (2022) 'Welcome to the world of the polycrisis', *Financial Times*, 28 October. Available at: www.ft.com/content/498398e7-11b1-494b-9cd3-6d669dc3de33

Vargas, R. (2024) 'Elon Musk on pace to become world's first trillionaire by 2027, report says', *The Guardian*, 8 September. Available at: www.theguardian.com/technology/article/2024/sep/07/elon-musk-first-trillionaire-2027

Varoufakis, Y. (2024) *Technofeudalism: what killed capitalism*. Brooklyn: Melville House.

Vince, G. (2022) 'The century of climate migration: why we need to plan for the great upheaval', *The Guardian*, 18 August. Available at: www.theguardian.com/news/2022/aug/8/century-climate-crisis-migration-why-we-need-plan-great-upheaval

Waitzkin, H. (2023) ' "Post"-pandemic capitalism: reform or transform? comment on "ensuring global health equity in a post-pandemic economy" ', *International Journal of Health Policy and Management*, 12, p. 7936. Available at: https://doi.org/10.34172/ijhpm.2023.7936

WHO Council on the Economics of Health for All (2023) *Health for All: Transforming economies to deliver what matters*. Final report. Geneva: World Health Organization. Available at: www.who.int/publications /m/item/health-for-all--transforming-economies-to-deliver-what-matters

Wilkinson, A. and Fairhead, J. (2016) 'Comparison of social resistance to Ebola response in Sierra Leone and Guinea suggests explanations lie in political configurations not culture', *Critical Public Health*, 27(1), pp. 14–27. Available at: https://doi.org/10.1080/09581 596.2016.1252034

Wolf, M. (2023) *The crisis of democratic capitalism*. New York: Penguin Press.

World Health Organization (2021) *Health promotion glossary of terms 2021*. Technical document. Available at: www.who.int/publications/i/item/9789240038349

Index